EQUESTRIAN
PILATES
SCHOOLING FOR THE RIDER

EQUESTRIAN
PILATES
SCHOOLING FOR THE RIDER

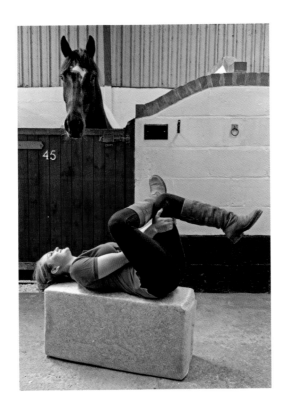

SUE GOULD-WRIGHT

J. A. ALLEN • LONDON

First published in 2015 by
J. A. Allen
Clerkenwell House
Clerkenwell Green
London ECIR OHT

J. A. Allen is an imprint of Robert Hale Limited
www.allenbooks.co.uk

ISBN: 978-1-908809-33-9

British Library Cataloguing in Publication Data
A catalogue record for this book is available from the British Library

Edited by Jane Lake
Design and typesetting by Paul Saunders
Photographs by Steve Holmes Photography
Line drawings by Jody Curtis

Printed by Craft Print International Ltd, Singapore

Disclaimer of Liability
The author and publisher shall have neither liability nor responsibility to any person
or entity with respect to any loss or damage caused or alleged to be caused directly or
indirectly by the information contained in this book. While the book is as accurate as
the author can make it, there may be errors, omissions, and inaccuracies.

CONTENTS

....

ACKNOWLEDGEMENTS

Without the support of my husband, Dave, I would not have had the time to develop my skills as an Equestrian Pilates instructor nor sit down and write this book. My family and friends' encouragement and belief in me have also been invaluable.

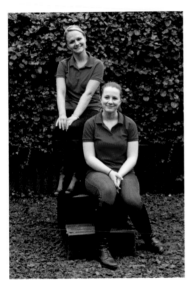

Fay and Christie

A huge thank you to my lovely models Christie, Fay, Jen, and Julia, and the horses of course, Jack, Onyx and my Ari – all of you were very well behaved and tolerant of my prodding and poking you into position!

Steve Holmes Photography for his patience and precision with the majority of the photographs herein.

A special thank you to Jody Curtis, for the wonderful illustrations; the poor girl had to decipher my desperate scribbles and annotations yet still managed to produce the fabulous images you will find within.

Without the stunning backdrop of Low Meadows Equestrian Centre, County Durham, the pictures may not have come out so well, so a huge thank you to the Bramwell-Dunn family for the use of the facilities.

Thank you to Lesley, from J. A. Allen Publishers, who has done a sterling job of nurturing, cajoling and advising me throughout the book development, and the rest of the team at J. A. Allen for producing such a superb book: Jane for patiently guiding me through the editing process, and Paul for the wonderful design work.

Thanks also to my riding instructors: Lucy Bramwell-Dunn with whom I have had many a happy lesson analysing and discussing the finest of tweaks of body position and aids, and Sylvia Loch and her beautiful horses for allowing me to experience the feeling of riding such sublimely schooled schoolmasters. Both have enhanced my riding, which in turn has developed my teaching.

And my wonderful, supportive clients who have been with me for many years and allow me to 'experiment' with mad ideas, teach me as much as I teach them and provide me with feedback week after week.

Finally, a special thank you to dear friends, Dorothy and Ron, who got me back in the saddle after many years away from horses and, best of all, allowed me to own my lovely equine soul mate, Arizona, who, although only a baby when we met, has taught me so, so much.

FOREWORD

....

BY KELLY MARKS

I'm a big fan of Pilates having used it with great effect to help the back issues that nearly all horse owners have, caused as much by mucking out and carrying hay bales than by actual riding I'm sure! Pilates not only helped ease the aches and pains but it also made me much more 'body aware'. This helped to avoid the bad posture that was causing the problem in the first place and I also felt it was of benefit to my riding.

I first met Sue when she came on an Intelligent Horsemanship course. Her well-rounded approach to horses and horsemanship, coupled with her Pilates training, makes her an ideal person to write this book. She truly understands the issues horse riders have, and uses her experience and training to resolve all manner of rider problems. Her knowledgeable approach, along with her 'do anywhere' exercises, will make this book indispensible to riders, especially those without access to a Pilates studio or class. Take this book down to your yard, put the exercises into practice and you'll soon be reaping the benefits. What's more, your horse will thank you for it.

KELLY MARKS
Founder of Intelligent Horsemanship

ABOUT THE AUTHOR

My name is Sue Gould-Wright and I am a pony-mad young girl trapped in a 40-something's body. I kiss my horse probably more than I kiss my husband, prefer to spend my days in muddy boots than pretty shoes and invariably smell more Eau de Cheval than Eau de Toilette. In other words, I am a perfectly typical horsey gal!

For as long as I can remember I have been sporty and carry many an old injury to prove it, yet thanks to Pilates I am still stronger, suppler, more flexible and body aware than I have ever been. As a result I move with my horse not against him; I 'feel' imbalances in him and in myself, and am able to isolate muscles to give the subtlest of aids; whispering to him not shouting.

I rode from the age of five until my early twenties when work took me away from horses for quite some time. With the exception of the odd hack out with friends or trekking on holiday I didn't really get back into the saddle until my mid-thirties.

During my break from riding I took up rowing. I loved being out on the water but suffered from recurrent lower back pain. My osteopath would sort me out but a few months down the line the pain would come back. In great pain one day I had to see a different osteopath as my usual one was away. There I was, in my twenties, quite shy, standing in my undies (the nice but not too fancy ones you reserve for such visits) being scrutinised by a handsome young Australian osteopath. I asked why my back pain kept coming back and when he gave me his answer I just wanted the ground to open up! His exact words were: 'You stand like a duck; you stick your backside out, your chest forward, your head forward and let your belly hang out. You need to do Pilates'. Thank goodness I had to lie with my face down for the next half an hour as I was crimson with embarrassment!

Having never heard of Pilates I did a bit of research and found a class and within weeks of attending my back pain had gone. It took a while to co-ordinate the postural corrections, breathing, and specific exercises but I was hooked.

So who am I to tell you how to get the most from your body? Well, after several years attending classes I had the opportunity to train as an Instructor with Body Control Pilates in London, qualifying in 2005. I have been a Pilates Instructor and Sports Massage Therapist for almost ten years, working with riders and ex-riders of all ages and abilities.

I have been around horses most of my life, fallen off a few and tried many disciplines both English and Western. I am also very, very normal and by 'normal' I mean that I have had my fair share of injuries and ailments – I can, quite literally, feel your pain and understand that most of us don't bend like we used to, if in fact we ever did to start with.

I teach throughout the UK, working with a very wide range of riders from top-flight competitors to those who just want to stay fit enough to get on, go for a ride, and get off again without aching for days!

I have my own gorgeous horse Ari, whom I have known since a yearling and had the privilege of being his 'Mum' since he was a three-year-old. We take it nice and easy, just enjoying each other's company with no deadlines doing whatever takes our fancy.

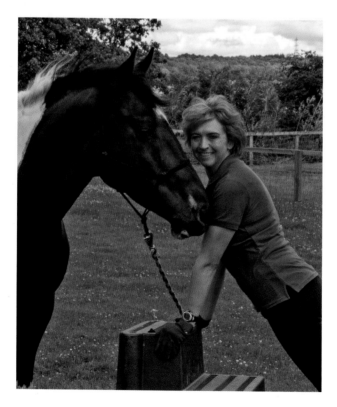

Ari helping with the cover shoot.

PRAISE FOR EQUESTRIAN PILATES

'As an endurance rider I spend long hours in the saddle. I have found Pilates very helpful in maintaining my flexibility. The work on strengthening my core helps me to stay straight and has improved my overall riding position.'

GILL BROWN

'I feel stronger, straighter and looser after every session. I am definitely a lighter, more balanced and confident rider since starting Pilates.'

JANE DAWSON

'Over the last few months Pilates has made me much more body aware, I walk taller, sit straighter and hopefully ride better with a deeper seat.'

JULIE STRAW

'I started Equestrian Pilates at the advice of my doctor after being diagnosed with arthritis in my lower spine. As most horsey girls know, back pain is part of the package, however mine had become quite severe and the 'doc' had me on so many pain killers I didn't know if I was coming or going half the time. Pilates has given me flexibility back, I haven't had a 'flare up' of severe pain for a long time, as when I feel it coming on instead of tensing up and going into spasm, I now deal with it with exercises and stretches I have learnt from Sue. I would highly recommend Pilates to anyone who suffers from any stiffness or aches whatsoever there are levels to help everyone.'

KAREN

'I would never have believed that it was possible to improve my riding by doing something other than riding. Pilates has really made a significant difference to my riding and all round posture.'

EILEEN DANIEL

INTRODUCTION

1

HOW EQUESTRIAN PILATES WILL HELP THE RIDER

Describing Pilates is one of the hardest parts of my work as an instructor, and when I talk to people about Equestrian Pilates I do sometimes get quizzical looks as people imagine how on earth they can get their horse on a gym ball or mat!

The Pilates method was created by Joseph Pilates and developed over many years by himself and his wife Clara, and thereafter by his students: the internet has many pages of information on Joseph for you to peruse so I shan't go into detail here. Pilates is a low-impact exercise method that is suitable for people of most age groups and levels of physical fitness and ability. The exercises are performed in a slow, controlled manner with the focus on the accuracy of movement rather than the number of repetitions. The exercises take the body through ranges of movement that we just don't do on a regular basis, for example, circling the arms around the body, circling the thigh bone in the hip socket or taking the back into extension.

Equestrian Pilates takes the general Pilates principles and applies them specifically to riders' needs, working on those areas that will enhance a rider's performance: the improvement of posture, mobility, flexibility, balance and core stability, learning how to use your body well and to be aware of when you are overusing it. We are also aiming for balance, not in the 'not falling over' sense but in the balance of the body itself: the back and front need to be balanced e.g. the back doesn't want to be tight and the front weak; both sides need to be balanced and equal so one side isn't tighter or stronger than the other.

The improvement of your posture will also be beneficial to groundwork with your horses, be that lungeing, long-reining, horse agility or natural horsemanship exercises. If you are aware of what your body is 'asking' the horse to do we can provide him with much clearer instruction. Whether you are riding or working from the ground, if you are not holding yourself well and using your body clearly you are asking the horse to decipher an aid from all of the 'white noise' you are producing. Examples include: the handler on the ground or the rider holding tension in the neck and shoulders, which could indicate to the horse that they are concerned about something, thus making the horse spooky too; an unbalanced rider using leg tension to stay on board, the horse has to decide which squeeze was an aid and which squeeze was the rider trying not to fall off! Another example is where imbalance causes a rider to balance with their hands; the legs may be asking for 'go' but the hands are saying 'whoa' – how is the horse to know which to react to?

Equestrian Pilates works to improve mobility and flexibility, particularly in the back and legs. When riding, your legs and seat are how you communicate with the horse; stiffness may cloud your conversations with your equine partner. The legs, hips and pelvis are also your suspension system when riding, absorbing the horse's movements and allowing you to become a more pleasurable cargo for the horse to carry.

Sadly, none of us are perfect in the old posture department, even me! But how does being a little bit crooked have an impact on your riding and your horse? If you are squint when sitting on your horse then the poor animal has to try to accommodate you, often resulting in him becoming crooked to match you. Your posture off the horse is unlikely to change greatly once you are sitting on the horse, so it stands to reason that you need to iron out any problem areas before you subject your poor, long-suffering equine to your tilts and imbalances.

Figure 1.1 shows some of the individual postural problems that we suffer from; however, in my experience there is never just one postural problem, and our bodies change day to day depending on what we have been doing.

If you take the example of the hollow-back posture on the top row (2), how would that rider look and feel? The rider's seat will be forward on their 'fork' (pubic bone), the lower back will be compressed, stiff and probably uncomfortable as it is unable to absorb the horse's movements, the shoulders will be rounded forwards and the head will be in front of the imaginary centre line of the body, which will cause balance issues.

If you then look at the images on the lower row you can see that most of them show a degree of weight shift to one side, which in the saddle could translate to more weight being on the seat bone on that side when

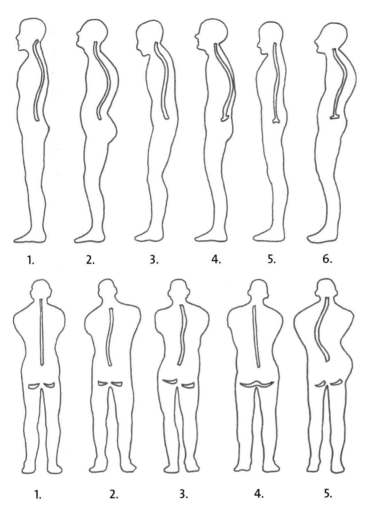

Figure 1.1 Standing postures

(top row): 1. correct posture; 2. hollow back; 3. flat pelvis; 4. slumping posture; 5. military posture; 6. round shoulders.

(bottom row) 1. correct; 2. high shoulder; 3. high hip; 4. head tilt; 5. severe scoliosis

you are sitting on the horse and a certain amount of shortening of the muscles between the underarm and the waist. Lopsidedness often takes more than a shift of weight from one seat bone to another to correct and so being told to 'sit to the left', for example, may just make you even more crooked; you always need to look at the bigger picture.

Looking at an alternative image (Figure 1.2), you can see that the various postural types have associated areas of muscle tightness or weakness, which will be addressed with the exercises in this book. But, before you tackle the exercises, go and find someone to take a photo of you from the side, front and behind so you know what you *actually* look like!

Once you start to think more about your posture and how you move, you will start to uncover what for me is the greatest benefit from Equestrian Pilates, that of much better **body awareness**: the more you think

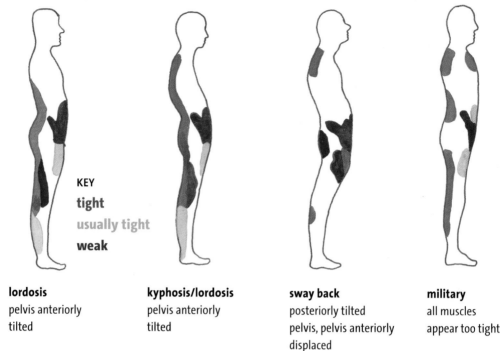

KEY
tight
usually tight
weak

lordosis
pelvis anteriorly
tilted

kyphosis/lordosis
pelvis anteriorly
tilted

sway back
posteriorly tilted
pelvis, pelvis anteriorly
displaced

military
all muscles
appear too tight

Figure 1.2 Posture types

about how you stand, sit, walk and ride the more you will find that you correct those old bad habits and create new good ones. Being lopsided will no longer feel normal, you will feel that it is inhibiting your fluidity of movement. With practice the ability to isolate movements from even the smallest part of your anatomy will have your horse and your riding instructor beaming with delight as you discover that elusive term **independent movement**, which, put simply, means that when you apply a leg aid you don't move everything from your ear lobes to your ankles too.

Having improved your posture and become enlightened in the dark arts of body awareness and independent movement, you need to move on to the fundamentals of Pilates: core stability and flowing movement.

Core stability is a term bandied about in the horsey world as the panacea for all riding faults. It is undoubtedly important, but the caveat to that is: *if it is done correctly*. I have been at events or on stable yards when people have said 'I don't need to do Pilates, I can hold the plank position for three minutes without breaking a sweat'. There is no doubt that the plank is a great strengthening exercise (again, when done correctly), I use it in my classes and can testify from the photo shoot that doing it for prolonged periods makes all of your abdominal muscles work; however, it is a static exercise. As a rider you need to practise engaging your core whilst performing movements because when you ride, even at walk, you need to stay balanced yet supple, i.e. to move freely, thus allowing the horse to move freely, for example allowing him to move your legs, seat and back with the swing of his ribcage.

The core needs to be working lightly all the time (Pilates teachers generally say about 25 per cent of the maximum core contraction, but more of that soon), and the correct muscles need to be working. What do I mean by that? Place one hand on your tummy below your belly button, the other hand above the belly button, now engage your core. Where do you feel the contraction; under your top hand? Did your shoulders lift? Did your backside clench? Did you hold your breath? If you answered yes to all these questions, don't panic; we will look in more detail at engaging your core *correctly* in the next chapter.

There are muscles in your body whose sole job is to act as stabilisers (your core muscles), others whose job is to mobilise your limbs and torso and some that actually do a bit of both. What can happen is sometimes muscles switch roles, they get either a tad lazy or over-excited, so you need to re-educate them.

Last in our line-up of Equestrian Pilates benefits comes **flowing movement**. By discovering your postural misdemeanours, improving your body awareness, independent movement and core engagement you can use the exercises in Chapter 3 to improve and maintain your flexibility and mobility.

THE BASICS

....

2

POSTURE

The main aim of developing great posture is not just about looking good, it is about holding your body in neutral positions whenever possible. So what does this actually mean? 'Neutral' is where your joints are in a position/state whereby there is minimal strain and misalignment, in and out of the saddle. (Figure 2.1) This figure shows examples of poor and ideal postures. What needs to be worked on now is how you can learn to *feel* when you are in an ideal posture, starting from your feet and working upwards.

FEET

Firstly, feel how you currently stand, focusing on:

*   Where the weight is across your whole foot – on the heels, toes, inside edge? Do you stand the same way on each foot?

*   How wide apart your feet are.

*   What angle your feet like to go in – toes in, toes out, toes straight ahead?

When you have established how you normally stand, try the following exercise.

FOOT POSTURE EXERCISE

*   Ensure your feet are around a fist-distance apart and that they are ideally pointing straight forward. This is to help with the overall leg alignment, making sure the knee points straight ahead and the thigh bone sits in a neutral manner within the hip socket.

Figure 2.1 Good and bad posture.

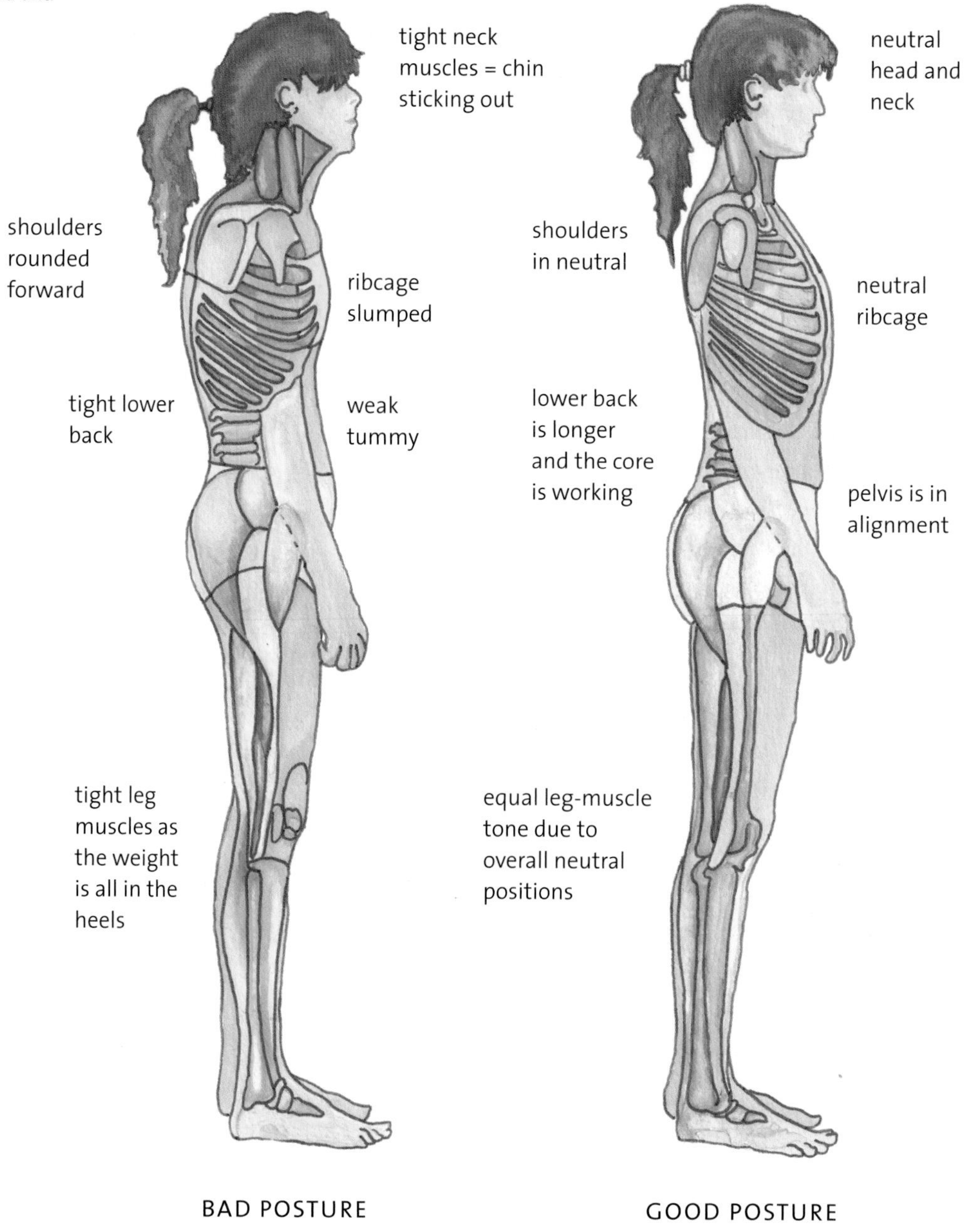

tight neck muscles = chin sticking out

neutral head and neck

shoulders rounded forward

shoulders in neutral

ribcage slumped

neutral ribcage

tight lower back

weak tummy

lower back is longer and the core is working

pelvis is in alignment

tight leg muscles as the weight is all in the heels

equal leg-muscle tone due to overall neutral positions

BAD POSTURE   GOOD POSTURE

- Feel your big toes pressing lightly into the floor; maintain that pressure and press the second, third, fourth and little toes down too.

- Feel the heels fully on the floor.

- Check the weight is evenly placed across the heels and toes, and evenly spread between both feet.

- Keeping that even pressure between the heels and toes, feel the outside edge of your foot pressing into the floor too, almost as if you were trying to slide your feet apart, but watch you don't lose the big toe pressure.

Having potentially changed just your foot posture how does the rest of your body feel? I would guess that you now have more engagement of your leg muscles and the muscles of your backside.

Find your inner child.
Get some paint and paper and both before and after doing the foot-posture exercise paint the bottoms of your feet and make footprints on the paper. Compare your before-and-after prints.

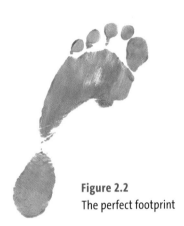

Figure 2.2
The perfect footprint

KNEES

Having worked on your foot position, your knees will probably be correctly aligned with the centre of the knee in line with the centre of the ankle; however, you need to ensure the knees are not locked, or hyper-extended to use the technical term.

I see many people whose natural tendency is to stand with their knees locked back, effectively bracing their legs. Many tell me they feel stronger and find it less tiring to stand like that but by working on the overall posture, this need to stand with knees pushed back should lessen.

By asking you not to lock your knees it does not mean that you need to stand with your knees bent like a downhill skier, just with a little softness in the knee joint. Why? Firstly, it is so much better for your knee joint to be held in a neutral, unforced manner because you are not compressing the joint capsule. Secondly, and probably more relevant to riders, you reduce the tension in the leg muscles, particularly the large muscles at the front of the thigh which are already well utilised in most riding disciplines.

PELVIS

A neutral pelvis is where, looking from the side, the hip bones and pubic bone are in alignment vertically. Sitting in the saddle, you will feel your two seat bones and, more lightly, your pubic bone in contact with the saddle.

The pelvis is generally held in one of three positions.

1. Butt sticking out (like a duck!) – the pubic bone is behind the hip bones (Photo 2.3a).

2. Butt tucked under – the pubic bone is in front of the hip bones (Photo 2.3b).

3. Neutral – pubic bone and hip bones are in alignment (Photo 2.3c).

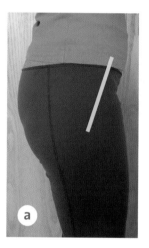 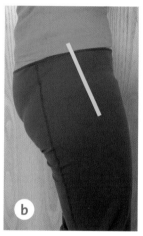 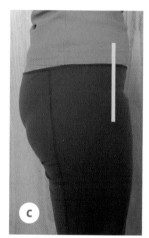

Photos 2.3a–c The three pelvic positions: a) the pubic bone is behind the hip bones. b) The pubic bone is in front of the hip bones. c) The pubic bone and hip bones are in alignment.

If you look again at the four postural positions described in Chapter 1 (see Figure 1.2) you will see the impact on tight/weak muscle groups in relation to these different pelvis positions. The most common one I come across is the backside-out position, or lordosis to give it its technical name, which leads to tightness and pain in the lower back, on and off the horse. A pelvis held out of neutral will generally either over-curve or flatten the lumbar spine and many people find that by correcting their pelvis position it has a very positive effect on their overall posture.

BACK

The back is so important in riding: it needs to be supple, strong and pain-free so that the rider can be moved freely by the horse's body, absorbing not blocking his movements.

You should aim to maintain your back in a neutral position so the centre of gravity stays roughly with that of the horse thus allowing him to move well, engage his core and lift his back. The art is to maintain the feeling of being upright with the correct curvatures in the spine without becoming tense and rigid. It is worth noting that the neutral spine shown in Photo 2.4 is relevant no matter what discipline you ride: yes, dressage and classical equitation benefit from a lengthened, elegant posture but neutral curves and a correctly working core will ensure you don't suffer discomfort when you are jumping or covering long distances in the saddle too.

Photo 2.4 shows Fay demonstrating the correct position of the spine:

- Lower back – curves inwards gently.

- Mid-back – curves outward to accommodate the ribcage.

- Neck – curves inwards gently.

Photo 2.4 The correct position of the spine.

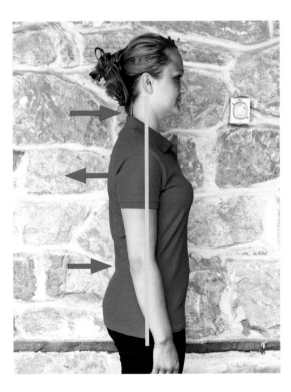

As mentioned above, by correctly positioning the pelvis the lower back should come naturally into a neutral position.

Feeling whether you have a correct back position is quite difficult initially; however practise with a mirror if you can, or ask someone to photograph you from the side, and take the time to *feel* how your back is when in the correct position.

Work on the following exercises to practise standing well with a neutral spine.

- Return to the steps for correcting the positions of your feet, knees and pelvis.

- Do you feel any discomfort in the lower back and/or an increase in pressure in the small of your back? If so, try to move your whole upper body forward slightly – imagine someone has a hand in the middle of your back and is pushing you lightly forwards while you hold your tummy in to prevent yourself from falling forwards onto your nose.

- For the mid-back you need to focus on your ribcage; imagine your ribcage contains a bell (Figure 2.5).

  If the bell is in neutral, your clapper (the bit that hangs in the bell and hits the sides to make the noise) will be hanging centrally and be still, making no noise at all.

  If your ribcage is lifted at the front, your chest will come upwards and your clapper will be clanging off your spine. (This lifted ribcage will also be shortening the muscles in your back making it tight and stiff.) To correct this lifted ribcage, be aware of the position of your breastbone and think about pressing the lower section of it lightly back towards your spine. Use your hands to feel if the bottom of your ribcage is lifted, and then imagine you are trying to slide the bottom of the ribcage into the waistband of your trousers, but only slightly or you will collapse and slump.

  Should you be slumped forwards with the bottom of the ribcage collapsed into your waistband and your clapper clanging off the tummy and ribs, start by thinking of the bottom of your breastbone lifting upwards and forwards gently but not too far or you will be clanging your bell the other way.

  It may also help to imagine you have a light shining from the lower section of the breastbone (see the dashed lines on Figure 2.5).

- Neutral – the light shines straight ahead.
- Ribcage lifted, over-arching your back – the light shines up in the air.
- Ribcage slumped – the light shines to the floor.

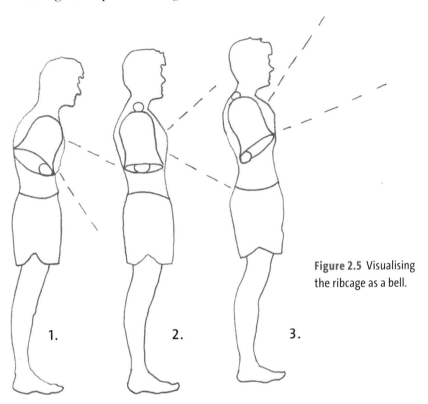

Figure 2.5 Visualising the ribcage as a bell.

1. 2. 3.

1. Ribcage slumped forward The bell clangs against the ribcage and the light shines down

2. Neutral ribcage
The bell is silent and the light shines straight ahead

3. Ribcage lifted upwards
The bell clangs against the back and the light shines up

- The final section of your spine to think about is your neck which, like your lower back, naturally curves slightly inwards. Your head, balancing on top of the spine, is usually what alters this natural curve. Allowing the chin to poke forward will deepen the neck curve, compressing some of the vertebral joints in the neck.

  To check your neck posture, place your hand on the back of the neck and feel if there are any small areas which feel they aren't in contact with your hand or feel over-curved.

When walking around, sitting at your computer, driving and riding you can regularly think about gently drawing your chin back towards your throat or if you are wearing a shirt, think of pressing the neck lightly back into the collar.

At the same time you are thinking of a light backwards pressure through the neck, ensure you are also aware of stretching slightly upwards through your spine. Quite often when asking clients to 'sit tall' or 'lengthen up' through their spine the natural reaction is to lift the chin – undoing all the good work you have just done – so try to think of the stretching-up coming from the centre of your head, or even as if someone is lightly holding the tops of your ears and stretching you up from there!

CORE STABILITY

To support your newly found ideal standing/riding posture you have to ensure your core stability muscles are working correctly. We are often told to engage our core but very rarely are we told how to do this. When working with new clients it is quite normal for me to see them pull in the whole of the stomach area, clench their buttocks, lift their shoulders up and hold their breath (all at the same time) when I ask them to engage their core. Knowing where these core stability muscles are located and then learning how to engage them in isolation is so important.

The main muscle you need to focus on is the transversus abdominis (Figure 2.6). I would like you to really feel how much of your torso this muscle protects and supports so, if it is not embarrassing to do so (you may be reading this in a public place after all), feel for the highest part of your ribcage at the front, now follow the curve of your ribcage all the way down and then round to where it meets your spine. Now, move your fingers down your spine to where it joins the pelvis, follow the rim of the pelvis all the way round to your hip bones and then down and round to your pubic bone. Pretty much all of the area within those bony landmarks is encompassed, underneath some other soft tissues, by the transversus abdominis muscle.

We go into detail on the correct engagement of your transversus muscle in Chapter 3, meanwhile you could try this:

- Place one hand on the lower part of your stomach and the other hand above it (Photo 2.7).

- Imagine you have been told to engage your core. Can you feel anything under your hands? If so, where?

- Mentally scan through your body, checking for other areas you might have 'activated' inadvertently – e.g. shoulders, buttocks, jaw.

There are other muscles involved when you engage your core but they are triggered to work without you thinking about it; they include the multifidus muscles deep within the back and to an extent the pelvic floor.

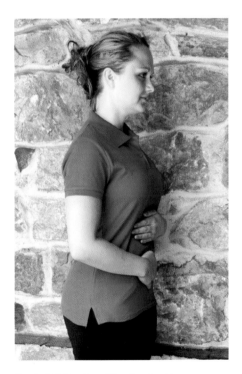

Photo 2.7 Hand position for checking your core engagement.

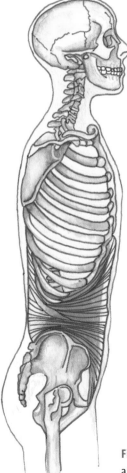

Figure 2.6 Transversus abdominis muscle.

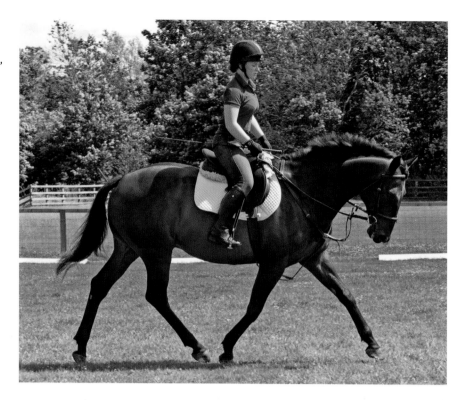

Photo 2.8 An efficiently working core is invaluable in your riding, helping you to be more in balance with your horse.

SHOULDER STABILITY

The shoulder joint is a ball-and-socket joint. To envisage how that looks, make a fist with your left hand and then cup your right hand over your fist. If you now start to move your fist around on the palm of your right hand you will see that too much movement scoots the fist out of the supporting hand. This is not so different from the action of the shoulder socket, albeit that there are ligaments, tendons, joint capsules and muscles to prevent the arm from pinging out of place, but work still needs to be done on making the joint as stable as possible as it is a shallow joint and therefore prone to injury.

By working on the stability of the joint, your shoulder posture will also be improved, specifically the common occurrences of shoulders rounding forwards and creeping up towards your ears (especially when you are concentrating on something else).

The following simple exercise, performed sitting or standing, will help you to find your shoulder-stabilising muscles and, if done regularly, help to tone them and make shoulder stabilising a subconscious act.

- Shrug your shoulders up and down becoming aware of where your shoulder blades are.

- Shrug your shoulders up towards your ears, think about where the outside edge of your shoulder blades are and try to use your back muscles to pull just those areas down towards your waist.

- Check that you haven't allowed your ribcage to lift up at the front resulting in you excessively hollowing your lower back.

- Again, raise your shoulders up and now, in addition to thinking about the outside of your shoulder blades drawing down, add the feeling of drawing your underarms down towards your waist too.

Can you feel how strong and stable this makes you?

Not only is shoulder stability and position important from a postural and aesthetic perspective but it will be invaluable in your leading and riding. If you hold on to the end of a lead rope and ask someone to pull against you (not too vigorously as you don't want to be injured) you will feel that if you only use your arms to resist you stand no chance, but if you engage your shoulder stabilisers not only will you be stronger but you will be able to apply a consistent pressure down the rope, which is a much nicer feeling for your horse.

This is also applicable to rein aids: by utilising your back muscles as discussed above you can send quiet, soft messages down the rein.

BREATHING CORRECTLY

You may be confused as to why I have included a section that tells you how to breathe; we do it day in, day out and so what could be more intuitive?

We do all breathe but how many of us breathe as efficiently as we could? When nervous or concentrating we are all prone to rapid, shallow breathing or just plain holding our breath completely.

'Lateral breathing' is a technique that is used a lot in Pilates and yoga. It teaches you to use your full lung capacity and to think about *where* in your lungs you are aiming your breath.

Find a scarf (or tail bandage/lead rope/pair of tights) and wrap it around your ribcage as shown (Photo 2.9). Take a breath in and feel which part of you moved: the top of the ribcage; the tummy? When clients do this exercise, as they take a breath in the tummy and chest often almost hollow inwards but, logically, when you breathe in, you are taking air into your lungs so the torso should expand outwards. The hollowing inwards is an example of how we can breathe poorly.

When you breathe in correctly, your diaphragm is pressed downwards as the lungs fill with air. Your ribcage should expand outwards. Wrap the scarf around your ribcage once more and taking a breath in try to push the scarf outwards to the sides – lateral breathing. You want to feel that you are actively aiming the breath into the bottom, outside corners of your lungs.

Your out-breath is almost an involuntary action; the diaphragm is a large muscle and once stretched when you breathe in, it will automatically recoil back into place, pushing the air out of the lungs as it does.

Don't try to do too many big in-breaths as you will get rather dizzy.

So why is breathing well or practising your breathing relevant to your riding or work with horses? Taking slow, deep breaths will help to lower

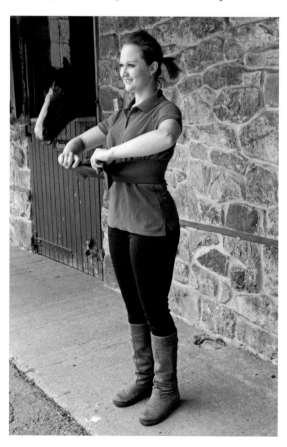

Photo 2.9 Band breathing. Fay is using an exercise stretch band, not a scarf, to do this exercise but note that her elbows are only this high so you can see where the band needs to be around the ribcage; hold your elbows in a more relaxed position down by your sides.

your heart rate and calm both you and your horse down in a tricky situation. My horse will halt or drop down a gait just from an out-breath. By breathing correctly you are taking more oxygen into your blood system, which is needed for muscle energy so if you are working hard, on or off the horse, you can increase your oxygen levels and decrease your carbon dioxide levels. I sometimes ask clients to try to breathe into a specific side of their ribcage if they are collapsing to that side on a circle or turn; the act of thinking about increasing the volume on that side of their torso helps to keep them centred.

A final note on breathing: if you have had any prior experience of Pilates you may have been asked to breathe in and out at specific points during an exercise. Whilst there are reasons for doing this, during the many years I have been teaching I have found clients new to Pilates become so focused on whether to breathe in or out that they end up doing the exercise itself, the movement of the body, so badly that it is counterproductive. To this end, I have not included specific breathing patterns with the exercises in Chapter 3 – but do promise not to hold your breath!

THE EXERCISES

3

BEFORE YOU BEGIN

As with all exercise, you need to make sure you are fit and well before commencing; if you are tired, sore or feeling unwell then please just read through the exercises with a cup of tea and try them another day. If you have any ongoing health issues please check with your doctor or other health professional before you begin.

I have not stated how many repetitions of each exercise to do: I would suggest no more than ten of each exercise would suffice, but if you find them hard, do fewer. Aim for doing fewer repetitions *correctly* than more repetitions incorrectly.

Standing Well

DEVELOPING A GOOD standing posture is the foundation for all the exercises in the following pages. By improving your posture off the horse, it will improve your posture and awareness in the saddle too. (Photos 3.1, 3.2 and 3.3)

● Ensure the weight is spread evenly across your feet, feeling the toes, heel and outside edge of your foot. The feet are positioned in parallel, about a fist-distance apart.

● The centre of the knee is in line with the second toe and the knee is soft, not pushed back.

● The pelvis is in neutral, with the hip bones and pubic bone in line when looked at from the side, and both hip bones are level with each other when viewed from the front.

● The lower back is softly curved and the ribcage is balanced centrally over the pelvis – the imaginary light on the front of the breastbone is shining straight ahead (see page 27).

● The shoulders are relaxed away from your ears, lightly drawing the shoulder blades down, and you should feel 'open' across your collarbones.

● The neck should be lengthened and slightly pressing back into the shirt collar with the head balanced beautifully on top!

● You want to feel that you are growing tall through the crown of your head but, at the same time, feeling grounded through your feet.

● Viewed from the side you would be able to draw a straight line starting at the tip of the ear, through the shoulder, centre of the ribcage, the hip, the knee and the ankle.

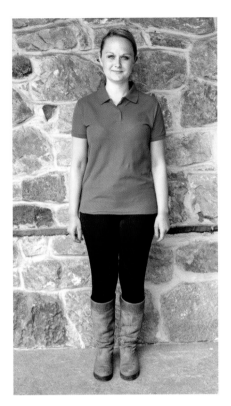

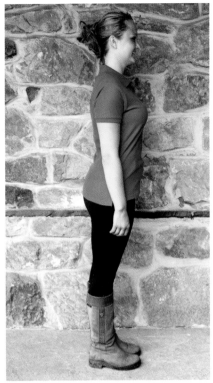

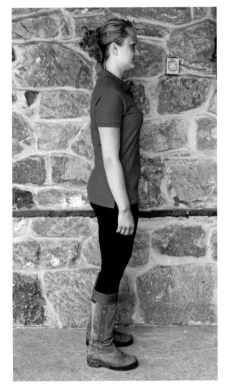

Photo 3.1 *above left* Fay demonstrating a lovely standing posture; note the hips and shoulders are level, although her left knee has a habit of sneaking forwards.

Photo 3.2 *above right* Fay is deliberately standing badly with her knees locked, backside sticking out and chest lifted.

Photo 3.3 *left* That's better; Fay is standing with the correct alignment.

Engaging Your Core

ENGAGING YOUR core correctly is the essence of improving everything: your balance, posture, mobility and even your breathing. Practising and perfecting this exercise from the ground will enable you to put it to great use in the saddle, helping you to stay secure but without tension, strong yet soft.

● Standing with one hand on the lower part of your stomach (remember, this is to help you engage the correct muscles) and the other hand above it, try to lightly pull your stomach muscles in away from the lower hand only. It should feel like the area below your tummy button is hollowing back towards the back waistband of your trousers. To help you engage the transversus abdominis muscle you may change from a flat hand on this lower part of your tummy to applying more pressure with your fingertips. This more precise pressure is great for waking up the transversus. Another useful tip for getting the correct muscles working is to think of this engagement as an inwards and upwards sensation, thinking of the area just above the pubic bone drawing inwards and upwards to the rear waistband of your trousers. Holding this engagement at only around 25–30 per cent of the maximum you can pull in, mentally scan through your whole body checking for areas you may have inadvertently activated. The usual problems are:
  · the shoulders have tensed and pulled up towards your ears;
  · the buttock muscles have clenched;
  · the tummy muscles under the top hand have pulled in – this is usually your 'six-pack' muscle, one that is used to move you rather than to support you;
  · you may also have tensed through your ribcage and held your breath.

● Once you feel you feel you have mastered engaging your core without other parts of your body joining in, still with hands in the positions discussed above, try walking around without losing the engagement of the tummy muscles. You should also be thinking about your lovely standing posture while you are walking, lengthening upwards with your whole body supple and relaxed.

● Photo 3.4 shows Fay deliberately engaging her core badly, incorporating all of the above mistakes. Photo 3.5 shows Fay correctly engaging her transversus muscle; note the relaxed neck and shoulders and how the body is back in correct alignment.

> **Tip** You can practise engaging your core, very discreetly, pretty much anywhere – sitting in the car or on the train, walking the dog, and obviously when you are riding. The more practice you put in the more refined your engagement will become.

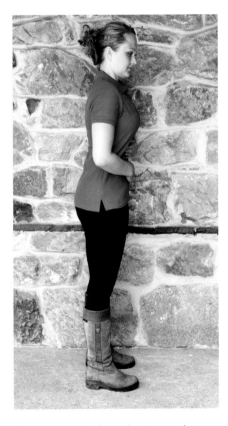

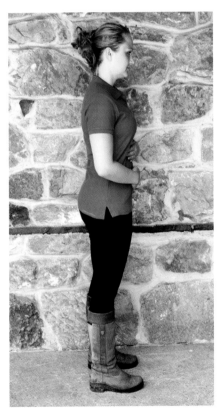

Photo 3.4 Fay deliberately engaging her core badly.

Photo 3.5 Fay engaging her core properly.

Rises and Pliés

THIS EXERCISE WILL challenge your stability and balance but is also great for improving your hip, knee and ankle mobility. It is a really useful exercise for your brain too as you have to concentrate on being relaxed, only engaging the parts of the body relevant to the exercise, and moving all at the same time – a bit like riding your horse.

- From your superb new standing posture, feel as though you are growing taller and taller through the crown of your head. Draw your lower stomach muscles (your core) in more and start to lift your heels off the ground until you are balanced on your toes. Keep the upper body still; try not to tip forwards or bend backwards from your waist. (Photo 3.6)

- Slowly begin to lower your heels down to the ground again. Try not to rock back onto your heels as you land, and keep those big toes firmly on the floor.

- With the core working well, and still with that feeling of lengthening upwards, you are going to bend at the hip, knee and ankle down into your plié position. (A plié is a classic ballet move when the knees are bent and the back is kept erect. The move has been utilised and adapted in Pilates and other workout forms.) As you bend, keep that alignment of ear, shoulder, centre of ribcage, hip and ankle – watch for your butt sticking out behind you. Heels stay on the ground. (Photo 3.7)

- Draw your core in and rise back to your start position.

> **Tip** To really keep that lovely lengthened feeling in your body, imagine someone is standing on a mounting block behind you and has the lower part of your head in their hands and is gently lifting you upwards, even as you plié down.

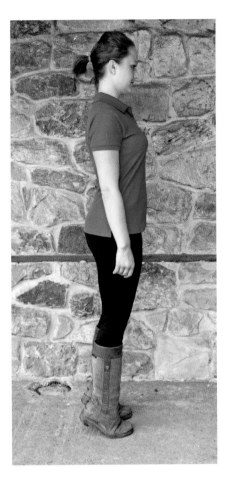 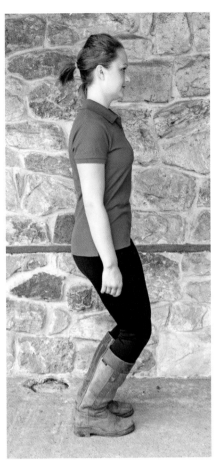

Photo 3.6 The rise: Fay has allowed her chest to lift a little, which you can see has hollowed her lower back slightly.

Photo 3.7 The plié: much nicer posture; well done Fay!

Single-Leg Rises and Pliés

THE EXERCISES

AS WITH THE DOUBLE-LEG version, this exercise will challenge your stability and balance and improve your hip, knee and ankle mobility but it will also help to identify, and go some way to correcting, any left/right imbalances in leg strength and mobility.

- You may want to stand near a doorway or wall as this exercise does require a bit more balance than you might think!

- Standing as for the Rises and Pliés exercise, take the weight onto your right foot, without tipping to the side. You can rest your fingertips on the wall lightly for support if you feel wobbly but try to just rest them there level with your side rather than gripping.

- Feel the weight evenly on your toes, heel and outside edge of the foot. Engage your core slightly more than for the double-leg version and focus on lengthening-up tall as you rise up onto your toes. Think of drawing your core up underneath your ribcage as you rise. (Photo 3.8)

- Slowly lower your foot to the ground, body in alignment, working your core to help keep you balanced. The more relaxed you can be, the easier this exercise will become, so stop tensing everything from your jaw to your toes.

- Still with the emphasis on maintaining a tall, lengthened torso, drop down into your plié. The centre of the knee should remain in line with the second toe (knees tend to wander out to the side or in to the centre as you bend), with the torso still in an upright, balanced position; make sure your buttocks are not sticking out. (Photo 3.9)

- Engage your core as you rise back up into your starting position and repeat on that side.

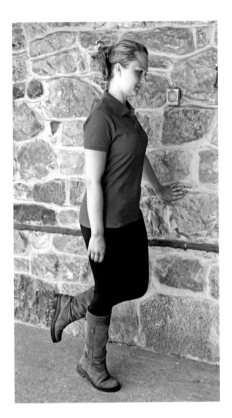

Photo 3.8 Single-leg rise

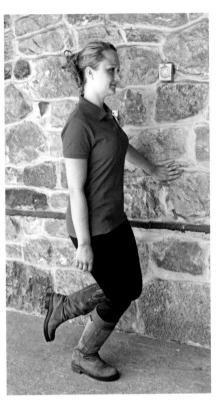

Photo 3.9 Single-leg plié

Pilates Stance

THIS EXERCISE WILL work different muscle groups in your legs from those you use standing normally, which will improve muscle tone in these areas.

- Standing with a neutral spine and pelvis, bring the inside edge of your heels together but have your feet in a V-position with approximately a fist-distance between the big toes, this will alter your leg position to one where the knees are pointing out to the sides slightly rather than forwards. Ideally you should feel that the *backs* of the legs are touching along their entire length. (Photo 3.10)

- Increase the sensation of pressing the *backs* of the thighs together, remember to keep the pressure the same along the whole length of the thigh. The area at the top of the thigh/lower part of the gluteal (backside) muscles (roughly where Fay's fingertips are in Photo 3.10) can become rather lazy, which results in the muscles losing tone and the wrong muscles taking over their role.

- Use your fingertips, in the same location as Fay has hers in the photo, to press lightly into the muscle as you try to rotate your thigh bones outwards a little more (just think knees pointing outwards) to increase the squeeze of the backs of the thighs. You should now focus on the very tops of the thighs and the bottom of the backside muscles working harder (where your fingers are). You do need to watch out that the *whole* of your backside hasn't squeezed though – we only want the lower area and the tops of the thighs working.

> **Tip** Try to notice if one of your buttocks starts working before the other. We all have a dominant side; we now need to learn to dominate *it* so that it behaves!

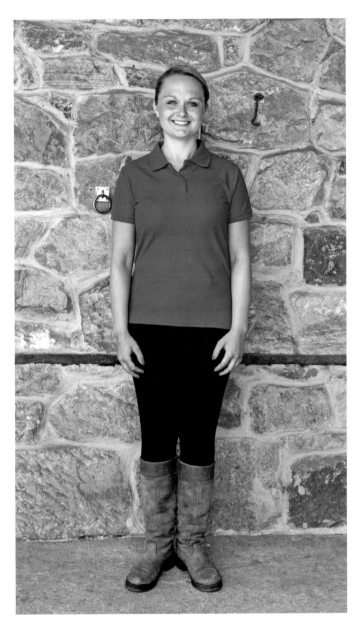

Photo 3.10 Pilates stance

Rises and Pliés in Pilates Stance

THIS EXERCISE WILL really get the deep leg and buttock muscles working during the rise and will stretch the inner thighs in the plié, all the while challenging your balance, stability and body awareness.

- Start in the Pilates-stance position with neutral spine and pelvis. Feel as though you are growing taller and taller through the crown of your head. Draw your lower stomach muscles (your core) in more and start to lift your heels off the ground, keeping the heels and legs firmly together, until you are balanced on your toes. Keep the upper body still, try not to tip forwards or bend backwards from your waist and keeps those legs together. (Photo 3.11)

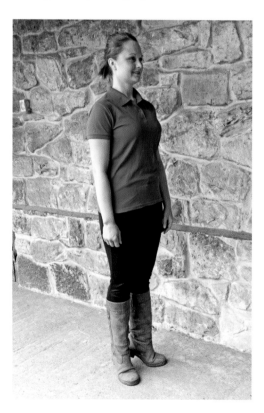

Photo 3.11 The rise in Pilates-stance position. Naughty Fay has locked her knees a little but, to be fair, we had left her up there for a while to get the photo.

- Keeping the heels touching, lower them to your start position with an upright spine and pelvis.

- Begin to drop down into your plié. As you plié keep the heels together and the whole foot on the floor; the knees will open to the sides stretching the inner thighs, calves and hips. Ensure the torso and pelvis stay in neutral; don't stick your backside out. (Photos 3.12 and 3.13)

- Now draw-in the core muscles and return to your starting position, squeezing the backs of the thighs together as you come up.

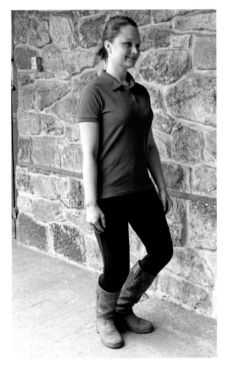

Photo 3.12 The plié in Pilates stance.

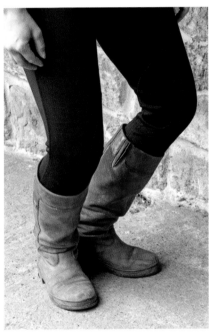

Photo 3.13 Close up of the plié position.

Tip The rise is the most challenging part of this exercise as the heels will likely come apart losing the connection of the thighs: imagine you are holding the money for your new saddle/horse/pair of boots between your thighs and if you drop it, you aren't allowed it back again – that should keep the legs working hard!

Standing on One Leg

THIS EXERCISE WILL develop independent movement of your legs while challenging your balance and stability, increasing your body awareness as you endeavour not to overwork through the rest of your body too.

● From your neutral standing position, place your hands on your hips and feel your whole body lengthening upwards, engaging your core up and under your ribcage.

● Feel the weight on your right foot evenly across the toes, heel and outside edge of your foot. Continue to lengthen up as you now slowly lift the left foot off the floor and slightly behind you. (Photo 3.14)

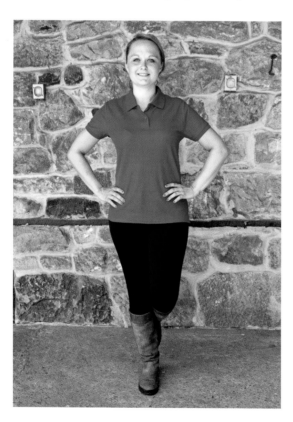

Photo 3.14 Standing on one leg. Try not to tuck your left foot behind you – that is cheating!

- As you lift the foot, be aware of your torso as your aim is to lift the foot *without any shift of weight* to the right. Keep the hip bones perfectly level; initially the tendency will be to hitch the left hip up slightly as you lift the foot from the floor.

- Lower the left foot to the floor, with no shift in weight from one side to the other and repeat the exercise to the right.

> **Tip** This is a great exercise for improving your overall body awareness as so many parts of your body want to join in! As I perform any exercise I mentally scan my body from top to toe, checking for areas of tension.

Standing Knee Fold

THIS EXERCISE WILL refine the independent movement of your legs with particular emphasis on keeping the pelvis still, which in turn will improve hip mobility. It will also challenge your balance and stability and improve your body awareness.

- From your neutral standing position, place your hands on your hips and feel your whole body lengthening upwards, engaging your core up and under your ribcage.

- Feel the weight on your right foot evenly across the toes, heel and outside edge of your foot. Continue to lengthen up as you now slowly lift the left leg upwards and in front of you until the knee is level with the centre of the hip, ideally, but if your hips are tight take the leg only as high as you can to keep everything in neutral. (Photos 3.15 and 3.16)

Photo 3.15 *right* Both hips and shoulders are staying nice and level.

Photo 3.16 *far right* Lovely side view of the knee fold showing Fay keeping her body and pelvis in neutral.

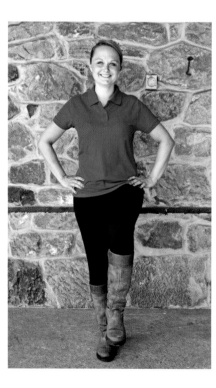
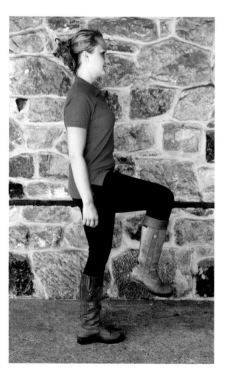

- Please check that as the knee has lifted, the pelvis has *not* tucked underneath you bringing your pubic bone forward and flattening the lower back; you need to keep the spine and pelvis in their neutral positions throughout. Also make sure that the hips have stayed level – your left hip may want to sneak upwards as the leg comes up.

  Also check that:
  - you are not holding your breath;
  - your shoulders haven't crept up to your ears;
  - your supporting knee hasn't locked back.

- As you lower the foot to the floor again, the body should stay still throughout with no shift of weight from side to side or front to back. (Photo 3.17)

- Change to the other leg and repeat the exercise.

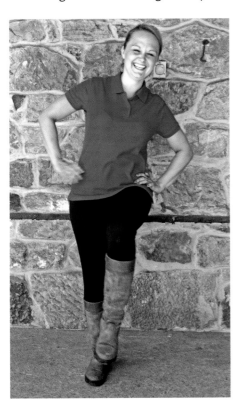

Photo 3.17 Whoops! This is what happens if you put your model off mid-exercise.

> **Tip** Try not to rush either part of the exercise. As a guide you could count 'one and two and three and four' to bring the leg up and repeat as you lower it.

Knee Opening

WITH THIS EXERCISE you again work on independent movement of the leg but there is an increased challenge to pelvic stability and body awareness as the leg not only lifts but also moves out to the side; great for fine-tuning awareness, balance, core strength, isolation and hip mobility.

- From your neutral standing position, place your hands on your hips and feel your whole body lengthening upwards, engaging your core up and under your ribcage.

- Feel the weight on your right foot evenly across the toes, heel and outside edge of your foot. Continue to lengthen up as you now slowly lift the left leg upwards and in front of you until the knee is level with the centre of the hip (Photo 3.18).

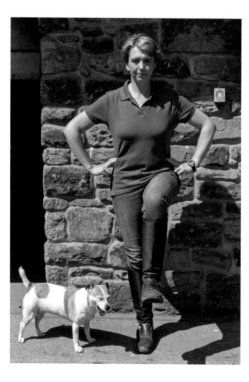

Photo 3.18 The starting position for your knee opening. (I can't decide if Pip, the yard dog, is bored or laughing!)

- Please check that as the knee has lifted, the pelvis hasn't tucked underneath you bringing your pubic bone forward and flattening the lower back; you need to keep the spine and pelvis in their neutral positions throughout. Also make sure that the hips have stayed level; your left hip may want to sneak upwards as the leg comes up.

    Also check that:
  - you are not holding your breath;
  - your shoulders haven't crept up to your ears;
  - your supporting knee hasn't 'locked' back.

- And now for the exercise! With your knee lifted, open the leg out to the side, keeping the knee as high as possible, ideally level with the centre of the hip socket (Photo 3.19). Be aware that as you open the leg to the side, the pelvis might want to move too, so keep the hips facing forwards all the time.

- Return the leg slowly to the centre and repeat the exercise several times without bringing the foot to the floor.

- Repeat with the other leg, making sure you are standing well before you start.

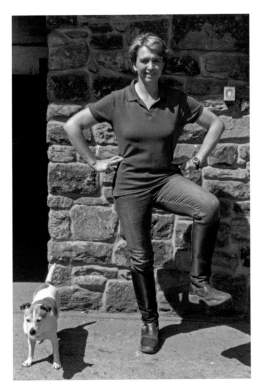

Photo 3.19 The knee opens to the side.

Tip This is a great exercise for warming up before you ride as not only does it loosen your hips but it also wakes up your body awareness and core.

Standing Oyster

THIS EXERCISE HELPS TO gently open and mobilise the hip joint. The support of the wall behind you will help to make you more aware of when other parts of your body move so that you may correct yourself, thus improving your body awareness to gain independent movement of the leg.

- Stand against a wall or door in your neutral standing posture. When you are standing in this position you will feel your backside touching the wall, your lower back will be slightly curved away, the mid-back will be in contact and your head will be very lightly in contact with the wall. The reason for standing this way is that the wall or door will then provide you with 'feedback' during the exercise, for example, if you twist your pelvis you will feel one buttock move away from the wall.

- Bend your right knee and place the sole of the right foot against the wall, knee pointing forwards (Photo 3.20). Now, keeping your pelvis completely still and level, open the right knee out to the side (Photo 3.21). Return it to the centre and repeat several times.

- Repeat to the left leg.

- This exercise may look rather easy but you need to focus on which parts of your body are moving when they should be still and relaxed, thus fine-tuning your independent movement of the leg. Usually areas that join in with the leg movement are the shoulders, which tense and lift, the back, which loses its neutral position, and the pelvis, which twists.

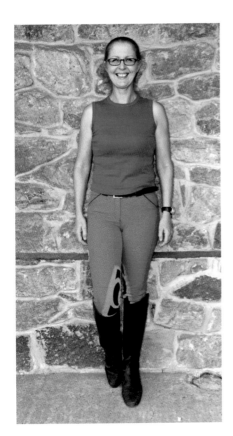

Photo 3.20 Oyster starting position

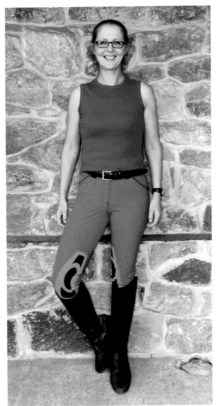

Photo 3.21 The leg opening out.

Tip Once you have mastered this against a wall, try it free-standing, without using the wall to give you feedback as to the unintentional movements you were making.

Zig-Zag

THIS EXERCISE IS A fantastic hip and ankle mobiliser which will also stretch the inside of the legs. Please remember to work at a level that is comfortable for you. As you repeat the exercise you may notice it becomes easier to do as muscles relax and stretch.

- Place a bale of shavings or hay near to the wall, close enough that when you lie down your lower leg will be parallel to the floor and your thighs will be upright with a 90 degree angle, roughly, at the knee and hip joints.

- Engage your core and ensure the back and pelvis remain in neutral throughout. Your feet are around a fist-distance apart and are flat on the wall (Photo 3.22a).

- Keeping the toes in position, rotate your legs so the heels go out to the sides (Photo 3.22b); keeping the heels in position, rotate the legs so the toes now go out to the sides (Photo 3.22c); continue to walk your feet outwards moving the toes and heels alternately.

- Once you have your legs as wide as you can manage, take a sneaky peak at your feet as you might find one is higher up the wall than the other (Photo 3.22d). (Fay didn't have that problem as Ari decided to correct her midway through the exercise.)

- Reverse the movements to walk the feet back to the start position and once there, again check the feet are level before you walk them out again.

> **Tip** You may find that when you walk the feet outwards the toes can swing out more than the heels and vice versa when walking them back in. If you do, to get the most benefit from this exercise try to challenge yourself to work harder at improving the stiffer, more difficult part of the movement and restrict how much movement you do of the easier part of the exercise.

THE EXERCISES

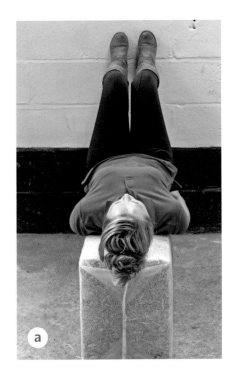

a

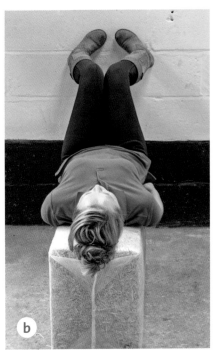

b

Photos 3.22a–d a) Zigzag starting position. b) Heels out: notice the movement is coming from the whole leg though. c) Toes out: Ari adjusting Fay's foot position. d) The final position, check your feet are level.

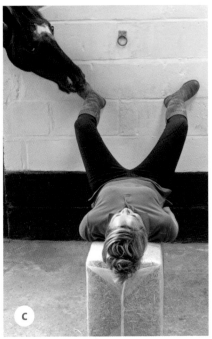

c

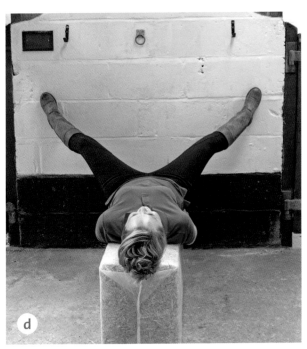

d

The Back Movements

HAVING A SUPPLE, mobile and pain-free back is very important for your riding, indeed every aspect of your life.

There are four ways your back moves:
1. Bending forward – flexion (Photo 3.23a)
2. Bending backwards – extension (Photo 3.23b)
3. Bending sideways – lateral flexion (Photo 3.23c)
4. Twisting round – rotation (Photo 3.23d)

● To keep your back as mobile as possible you need to move it in all four directions; however, you need to do this correctly, increasing your awareness of which parts of your back are stiff and tight and which parts are very mobile.

● There are generally three very mobile bits of your back: the lowest part of the back where the spine meets the pelvis, an area in the middle part of the back and the base of the neck (Photo 3.24). When we first start doing back-mobilising exercises we subconsciously want to move as far as possible. However, this often results in us really pushing into the bendy bits to compensate for the areas that are stiff. This can actually lead to us becoming sore in one or all of these three points of our backs.

● A lot of people have cameras on their phones and so if you are doing an exercise and are not sure how your back is moving ask someone to take a photo of you.

> **Tip** The main problem to watch for is when you are moving your spine in a forward flexion exercise – if your back looks hunched, particularly the mid to upper back, then you are probably trying too hard in that area. Aim for a smooth curve.

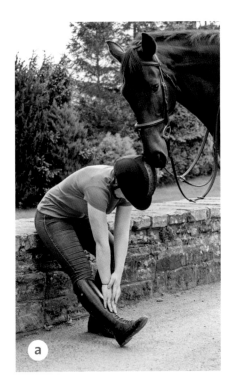

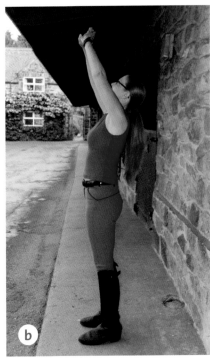

Photos 3.23a–d a) Flexion; b) extension; c) lateral flexion; d) rotation.

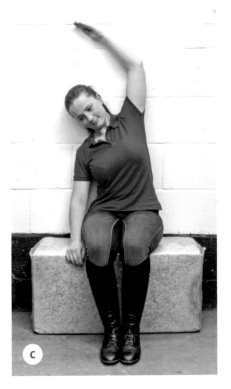

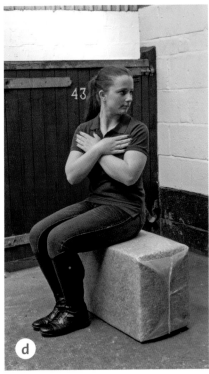

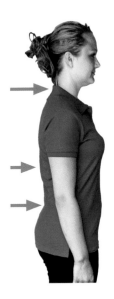

Photo 3.24 *above*
The three most mobile parts of your back.

Hamstring Studio Stretch

THE STUDIO STRETCHES are effective back-mobilisation exercises which, with practice, will develop your ability to isolate your spinal movements allowing your back to move as freely as possible through each joint. This hamstring version will also stretch the back of the thigh.

- Sit on a bale of hay or shavings with your back against a wall or door, place one leg out straight in front of you with the other foot resting on the floor. Your back will be in neutral so you will feel your buttocks against the wall, the lower back will either curve away from the wall slightly or may not be pressed as firmly into the wall as the rest of your back, the mid-back will be in contact with the wall and the neck will form another curve away from the wall. Your head/hair should just brush the wall lightly; if you push your head too far back you will cause tension in the neck. (Photo 3.25)

- The aim of this exercise is to move your spine one bone at a time until you have curved forwards with your back in a C-shape.

- Engage your core lightly, feel yourself growing taller and think of starting the movement from the crown of the head.

- Draw your chin lightly in towards your throat – this will tilt the head so the crown of the head is now pointing forwards and your neck has started to roll away from the wall. Starting from the base of the neck, one bone at a time, start to peel the remainder of your back away from the wall, engaging your core a little more with each movement, sliding your hands down the outstretched leg as you go. (Photo 3.26)

- You will reach a point where you start to feel a stretch down the back of the straight leg (the hamstrings); hold that stretch for a count of ten or longer if you feel comfortable doing so.

- **Please note** you should feel a comfortable stretch – never push yourself into pain. Also, how long to hold a stretch will differ from person to person.

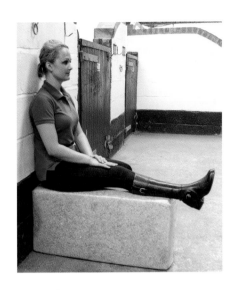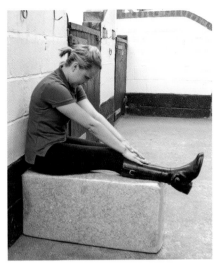

Photo 3.25 *far left*
The starting position for the Hamstring Studio Stretch.

Photo 3.26 *left*
Stretching forward, note the nice soft knee joint.

For the most benefit, hold the position until you feel the stretch ease, come out of the position for a count of three and then move back into the stretch – you should be able to get a little further.

- By doing this exercise sitting against a wall you can use the wall to help you feel how your back is moving when you roll forward and roll back up into the sitting position; this is what I mean by the wall providing you with feedback during various exercises. You may feel that one side of your back leaves the wall first as you roll forward which could indicate that the tummy muscles on that side are stronger and pulling that side more than the other. By taking the time to feel these little differences in how you move you are taking steps to correct and adapt your ingrained movement patterns.

- Start to roll back upright, starting the movement with a deeper engagement of the core muscles and rolling back up through the pelvis, lower back, mid-back, neck and head in sequence, again aiming for the sensation of moving one bone at a time.

- Repeat to the other side.

> **Tip** The backs of the legs are usually pretty tight so go into the movement carefully the first time. Once in the stretch, ensure you haven't held your breath and tensed your shoulders.

Long-Frog Studio Stretch

THIS STUDIO STRETCH will give more of a lower back stretch than the Hamstring Studio Stretch. By sitting with your feet together it may also stretch your hips and thighs, and by checking if your knees are level in both the start and stretched positions it will show you if one hip is tighter than the other.

- Sit on a bale of hay or shavings with your back against a wall or door, your feet together and your knees bent. Try to relax the leg muscles in this position; if your legs are tense you may not move as freely. Your back will be in neutral so you will feel your buttocks against the wall, the lower back will either curve away from the wall slightly or may not be pressed as firmly into the wall as the rest of your back, the mid-back will be in contact with the wall and the neck will form another curve away from the wall. Your head/hair should just brush the wall lightly; if you push your head too far back you will cause tension in the neck. (Photos 3.27a and b)

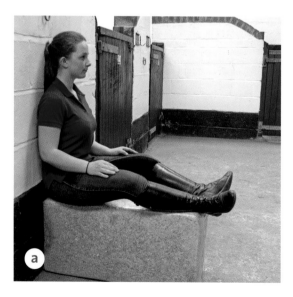 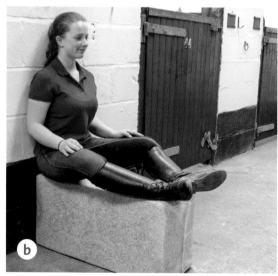

Photos 3.27a and b a) The starting position for the Long-frog Studio Stretch. b) The long-frog leg position.

- Engage your core lightly, feel yourself growing taller and think of starting the movement from the crown of the head. Again, the aim of this exercise is to move your spine one bone at a time until you have curved forwards with your back in a C-shape.

- Draw your chin lightly in towards your throat, this will tilt the head so the crown of the head is now pointing forwards and your neck has started to roll away from the wall. Starting from the base of the neck, one bone at a time, start to peel the remainder of your back away from the wall, engaging your core a little more with each movement, sliding your hands down your legs until you feel a stretch in the lower back/buttock area. (Photo 3.28)

- Hold this stretched position for at least a count of five, trying to relax your shoulders, back, hips and legs as you do so. It may be helpful to take a couple of nice, big breaths in and out while you are stretching forwards: breathe in, and concentrate on releasing muscle tension/relaxing every time you breathe out.

- Start to roll back upright, starting the movement with a deeper engagement of the core muscles and rolling back up through the pelvis, lower back, mid-back, neck and head in sequence, again aiming for the sensation of moving one bone at a time.

Tip Once you have moved into your stretch look at the level of your knees – are they even? How far down do they drop? If one knee is higher than the other this indicates a tighter hip; you can now work on releasing it using the hip exercises.

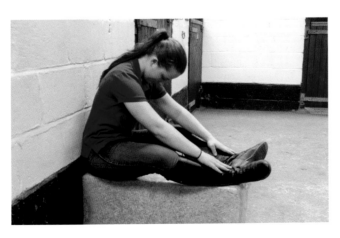

Photo 3.28 Curving down into the stretch; notice how even and flexible Christie's hips and knees are.

Seated Rolldown with Hamstring Stretch

THIS IS ANOTHER GREAT back mobilising exercise with a stretch to the back of the leg too. As you are not sitting with your back against a wall as in previous exercises, you will really have to feel how your back is moving – a good challenge for your body awareness.

● Sit on the edge of a bale of shavings or hay, or a chair. Feel the weight is even on both seat bones as you straighten one leg in front of you, keeping the ankle, knee and hip in alignment (Photo 3.29). Sit tall, engage your core lightly and start to nod the head, drawing the chin slightly back towards the throat.

● Starting with your neck, start to roll down through your spine one bone at a time keeping the weight even on your seat bones. The hands slide down

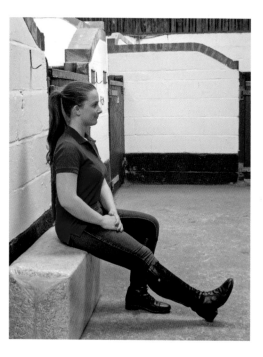

Photo 3.29 The starting position for the Seated Rolldown with Hamstring Stretch, note Christie's lovely neutral position.

the leg at the same time until you feel a stretch in the back of the thigh. Do take care not to push the knee back, though. (Photos 3.30a and b)

- It is worth mentioning for those of you with very mobile lower backs that you are trying to curve your spine down, drawing your tummy in as if rolling over the top of something (a beach ball for example); do not try to get your chest onto your leg as some clients like to do.

- Hold the stretch for as long as is comfortable and, starting with the pelvis, roll back up into an upright position, one bone at a time as if you are stacking little building blocks one on top of another. As you roll up, make sure the weight stays even on your seat bones throughout.

- Repeat to the other leg.

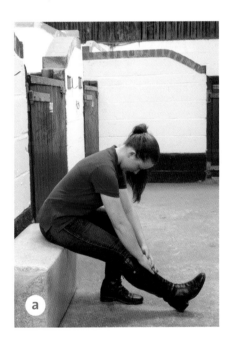 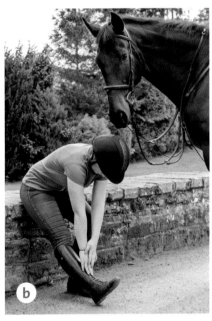

Photos 3.30a and b
a) A nice even curve through the whole back;
b) This exercise is a great warm up before a ride.

Tip If you don't feel much of a stretch in the back of the thigh, try lightly bending the ankle so the toes come in towards you. This will also give you a calf stretch.

Standing Rolldown

THIS STANDING VERSION of the Rolldown is another great back mobilising exercise and with only your feet in contact with a surface it will really challenge your body awareness and balance and *should* be more work for your core.

- Standing correctly with your feet roughly a fist-distance apart, feel you are lengthening upwards through your entire spine whilst maintaining a grounded feeling through your feet. (Photo 3.31) Lightly engage your core and nod your head, bringing your chin slightly back and in towards your throat.

- Start to roll your back down beginning from the neck and trying to move each vertebra individually. Mentally break the movement down, engaging your core slightly more the further down the movement you get.

  1. Roll through your neck (This very subtle curve in the neck is shown in the photo for point 2).

  2. Imagine there is a tall fence roughly level with the middle of your chest; you need to curve through your upper back to roll over the top of it (the thought of wine and chocolate on the other side of the fence motivates me!) (Photo 3.32a)

  3. Roll the lower back but try to keep the pelvis upright (Photo 3.32b).

  4. Finally allow the pelvis to tilt and roll down as far as you comfortably can (Photos 3.32c and d).

- As you roll, keep the head and neck curved so that you look at your stomach and then thighs as you move further and further down. The temptation will be to look at the floor but this action actually curves your neck into an extended not flexed position. The arms should be hanging down, relaxed and floppy, as Jen demonstrates in the photographs.

- Keep the weight even over the entire surface of both feet as you roll. The first time you do this exercise your weight might shoot back into your heels, which will have the knock-on effect of you sticking your backside

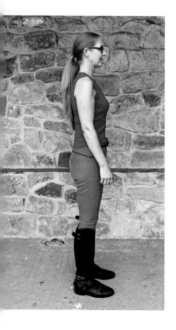

Photo 3.31 Jen in a lovely neutral standing position.

right out behind you. All through the Rolldown you should aim to keep the legs upright, although you are allowed to bend the knee slightly if the backs of the legs are screaming!

- To reverse the exercise you will need to engage your core strongly to role the pelvis into an upright position without the backside pushing back – if you feel the weight staying consistently even over the whole surface of your feet this will give you valuable feedback: if the weight moves back into your heels your backside will be sticking out behind you. Then keep working the core well as you roll through the lower, mid and then upper back until you have returned to a tall, lengthened standing position.

Tip If you have a tight lower back, try standing with your back against a door or smooth wall with your feet about one foot's distance away from the wall. Keeping your knees bent forwards roll down using the wall as feedback that you are moving evenly, for example if one side of the back leaves the wall before the other. When you roll up again, the wall is also a great tool for really trying to move sequentially through your spine.

Photos 3.32a–d *photos below*
a) Movements 1 and 2: the subtle roll through the neck and rolling the upper back. b) Movement 3: the pelvis stays upright. Movement 4: c) Rolling the pelvis and d) Jen has rolled as far as she comfortably can, note though that she has just started to lose the vertical alignment of hip/knee/ankle slightly.

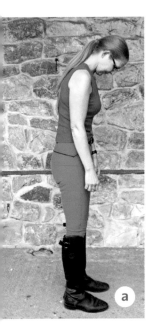
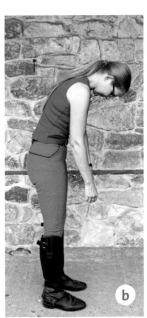
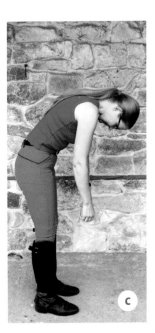
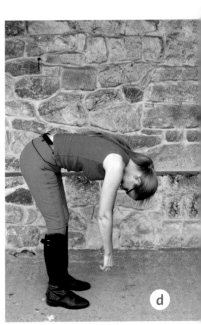

a) b) c) d)

Seated Side Reach

THIS EXERCISE WILL laterally (sideways) flex the spine which, along with the other back exercises, will help to keep your back as flexible as possible. It also stretches the sides of the body and the arms.

- Sit with your back against a door or wall. Feel the neutral curves in your spine as you sit there: the lower back curves slightly away from the wall or has a lighter pressure on the wall than the mid-back which will be firmly in contact, the neck curves slightly away from the wall and the head/hair lightly brush the wall.

- Take your arm out to your side, palm facing inwards. Engage your core. Ensuring the shoulders stay away from your ears, lengthen up tall and then start to stretch the arm up and over your head (Photos 3.33a and b). Ideally the distance between your ear and your arm should stay the same throughout the stretch (initially your arm may decide it just wants to flop over your head which is wrong – you need to keep that distance). If you were in a studio I would say aim the fingertips to where the ceiling meets the wall to ensure that throughout the stretch you are feeling that 'upwards' sensation.

- As you return the arm and body to the start position, continue to feel that you are lengthening upwards the entire time, almost as if you are lifting the ribcage away from the waist throughout.

- Repeat to the other arm.

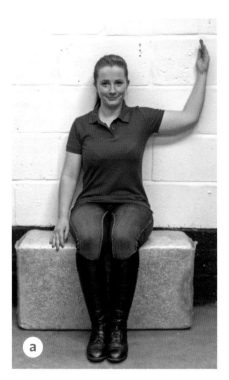
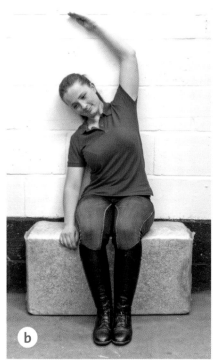

Photos 3.33a and b a) The arm is raised ready to move the torso into the side bend.
b) A lovely side bend from Christie.

Seated Rotation

Rotation is great for mobilising your back and finding (and releasing) your stiffer side.

- Sitting on a bale or chair, your feet are firmly on the floor and your seat is evenly weighted over both seat bones. Cross your arms over your chest as shown. (Photo 3.34a)

- Just moving the head and neck to begin with, turn to look over your left shoulder. Now, keeping the weight even on your seat, engage your core and start to turn through your spine to look further behind you (Photos 3.34b and c). Ensure the weight is still even over your feet and your seat as you have turned, no rolling onto the back pockets of your trousers or tilting to one seat bone. Hold that position for a count of five, checking as you do that the shoulders are even and away from your ears and that you haven't collapsed and shortened between underarm and waist.

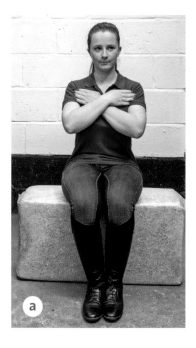
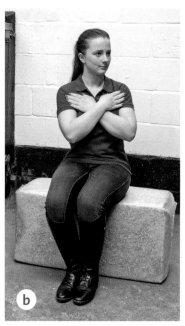
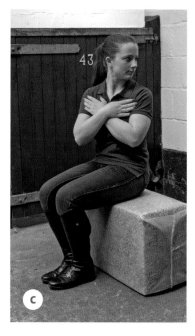

- Return to the starting position by engaging your core and reversing the movement this time starting with the lowest part of your back and finishing with the head and neck.

- Repeat to the right.

- You can also do this exercise in the saddle as a warm-up but don't cross your arms; keep the reins in one hand as you rotate. If your horse is responsive to seat and weight aids he will soon tell you if your weight shifts and/or you tilt to one seat bone as he will go off in the direction your shift asked for.

> **Tip** Imagine you have a thin pole against your back (or find a fence post to lean against) and, as you rotate round, keep your back in contact with the post to ensure you don't shift your weight to one side.

◀ **Photos 3.34a–c** *opposite page*
a) Rotation starting position with the shoulders nice and relaxed. b) Notice the rotation is starting from the top of the spine. c) A lovely, even rotation with the legs staying in their starting position.

Seated Bowman

A LOVELY EXERCISE TO mobilise your spine by using rotational movement; with the arms away from your sides this time it will challenge your body awareness too.

You are going to rotate your torso as with the Seated Rotation exercise but the arms are not in contact with your body so you will not have that feedback of how your body is moving (tilting to one side, for example) under your arms – great for your body awareness!

- Sitting on a bale or chair ensure the weight is centred over your seat bones and your feet are firmly and evenly placed on the floor. Hold your arms out in front of you, palms down, slightly wider than shoulder width apart making sure the shoulders are relaxed and away from your ears. (Photo 3.35a)

- Leading with the left elbow, start to draw the left arm back bending it as it comes level with your side (Photo 3.35b). As the arm is moving, engage your core and begin to turn through the head and neck and then begin to straighten the arm stretching it behind you; turning your body as far as you can, keep the weight even over your seat (Photo 3.35c).

- Hold that position for a moment, stretching both arms in opposite directions. As you hold, scan through your body checking for areas of tension (particularly the shoulders) and imbalance (have you rolled onto one seat bone or curved your buttocks underneath you?). Reverse the movement to return the arms and torso to the start position.

- Repeat to the other side.

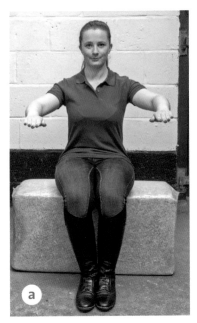

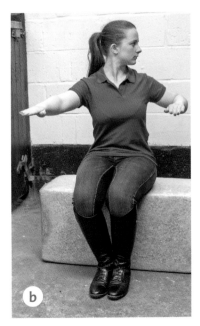

Photos 3.35a–c a) The arms are held out in front, palms down, with the shoulders relaxed, and a feeling of 'openness' across the chest. b) The start of the rotation; the left elbow is the perfect height. c) The end position; notice how much core work Christie is doing to maintain her strong position.

Photo 3.36 *below* When mounted, don't do this exercise with both hands without helpers.

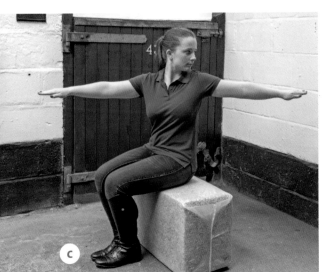

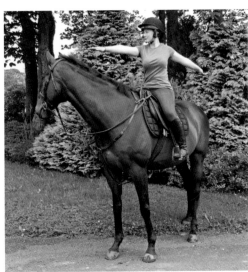

Tip This is such a good exercise for mobilising your back but it is also a great tool for becoming aware of where your body likes to 'cheat', i.e. do you tilt to one side as you turn, roll onto the back pockets of your trousers instead of staying even on your seat bones? You can do this in the saddle too but I suggest holding the reins in one hand – Christie did it with both hands here but there were three of us on standby to catch Jack if he decided to wander off. (Photo 3.36)

Standing Side Reach

THIS STANDING VERSION of the lateral flexion/side bend exercise really helps to open up all the small joints in your spine and has an added stretch to the outside of the hip compared to the Seated Side Reach.

- Stand an arm's distance away from a stable door, or something sturdy you can hang on to. Holding on to the door, bring your outside foot in front of the inside foot as shown. Keeping the shoulders relaxed and away from the ears, take your outside arm out to the side and, turning the palm inwards, raise it upwards. (Photo 3.37)

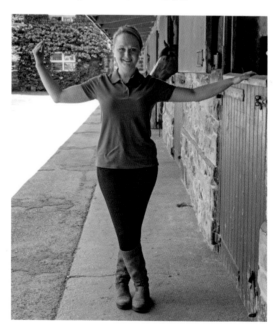

Photo 3.37 The outside foot has crossed in front of the inside foot and the outside arm has been raised.

- Keeping the distance between the ear and the raised arm the same throughout, engage your core and ensure your hips are facing forwards as you start to lengthen upwards and bend sideways towards the door, starting the movement with the ear dropping to the shoulder. You should feel a stretch down the side of your body.

- Still lengthening the whole body in your side-bend position push the outside hip outwards, hanging off the hand on the door (Photo 3.38). In addition to the stretch in the torso you should now feel a stretch on the outside of the hip and leg.

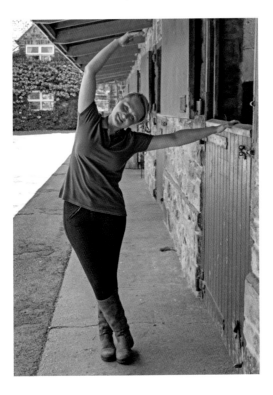

Photo 3.38 Really push the outside hip away from the door.

- Return to the start position, lengthening through your whole body as you do – don't slump!

> **Tip** As you have brought one foot across the other, the hips may become a little wayward and want to twist, so make sure at every point in the exercise that the hip bones both face forwards. The outside one is likely to sneak forwards if you are quite tight in the hip and thigh.

Spine Curls – Feet on Wall

THIS GENTLE mobilisation exercise for the whole back is a favourite of mine. Having your feet up on the wall really helps to increase the stretch, particularly in the lower back.

- Lie on a bale, or bales (if you feel unsafe, you could even lie on the floor) with your feet flat on the wall. Your legs want to be positioned so that your thigh bones are vertical and your lower legs are parallel to the floor. Your back and pelvis are in neutral and your core is lightly engaged, arms are down by your sides, holding the bottom of the bale for support. (Photo 3.39a)

- You are aiming to move your spine one bone at a time into a nice, deep C-curve while keeping your head still and shoulders relaxed.

- Engage your core slightly more and think of tilting your pelvis so that your lower back comes down onto the bale. (If your lower back was already touching the bale go back to the start position and check that your legs are far enough away from the wall and/or that you hadn't just forgotten about your pelvis position!)

- With your pelvis tilted, start to send the knees upwards, your buttocks will start to lift off the bale but you need to think about your back moving one bone at a time. Imagine that I have my arm across the lower part of your ribcage and that you are curling up and under it – this will stop you flattening your back and thrusting your chest upwards. (Photos 3.39b and c)

- Depending on your ankle/boot flexibility your heels may lift off the wall as your back lifts, that is fine.

- Reverse the movement, feeling for the highest part of your back that is off the bale and rolling down, one bone at a time, from that area.

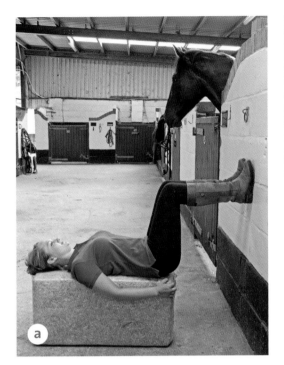

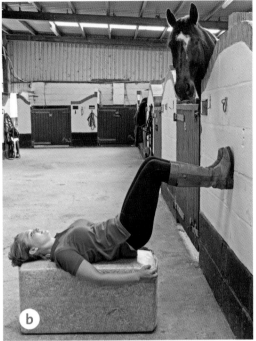

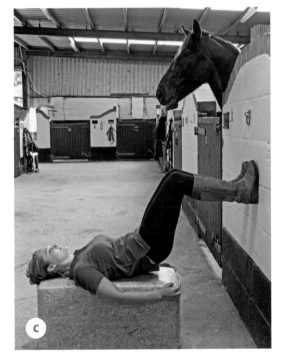

Photos 3.39a–c a) A good starting position for the Spine Curls. b) A nice even C-curve through the lower back. c) Note the core working to keep the breastbone heavy to maintain the up-and-under curl.

Tip If you feel like you are pushing yourself headfirst off the bale you need to engage your core and buttock muscles a little more and focus on the knees leading the movement, not pushing with the feet to obtain the lift in the back.

Standing Threading the Needle

THIS IS ANOTHER lovely mobilisation exercise for your back using rotation; rotation helps to keep the smaller (facet) joints in your spine moving freely, which in turn improves your general back flexibility.

- Stand facing a wall or door with your hands on the wall in front of you, slightly lower than shoulder height. Make sure you are standing just less than your arm's length away from the wall, you don't want to be too close or far away. Your torso and pelvis are in neutral and your core is working lightly. (Photo 3.40a)

- Take your left hand off the wall and turn it so that the palm faces you. Keeping the back of the left hand quite close to the wall, start to move the hand to the right, taking it just underneath the right wrist. (Photo 3.40b)

- As you have started to move the arm your body will have begun to turn: make sure that your hips stay still as the turn should come only from the torso/spine. (Photo 3.40c)

- Stretch as far as you feel you can, engaging your core a little more as you move further round. Check that you haven't stuck your backside out!

- Reverse the arm movement and replace your left hand on the wall.

- Repeat to the other side.

> **Tip** To feel if your hips are moving, take your attention down to your feet – if your hips/pelvis have moved the weight will no longer be even on your feet. You could also just have a glance down!

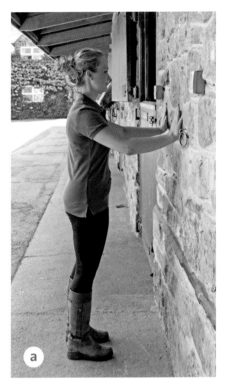

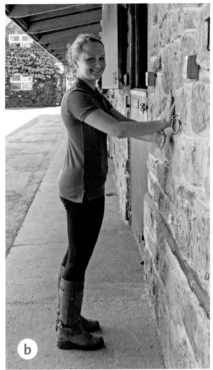

Photos 3.40a–c a) A lovely neutral starting position. b) The arm begins to move through, the body rotating. c) Note that the legs and pelvis have remained still to get the rotation of the spine; the rotation is not coming from the legs.

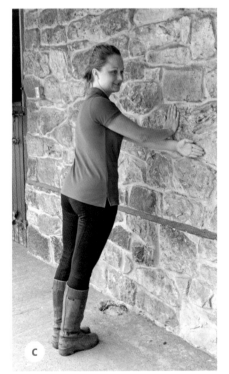

Lying Hip Rolls

THIS IS A GREAT exercise to help keep the lower back supple. It is a rotation exercise but, unlike the previous exercises, the rotation starts in the base of the spine rather than the neck.

- Lying on a bale with your spine and pelvis in neutral, core working lightly, place your feet on the wall. You should ideally have a 90 degree bend at the hips and knees so the bale should be approximately the length of your lower leg away from the wall. The lower leg is parallel to the floor, thigh bones are pointing straight upwards. Your hands are holding the end of the bale lightly. (Photo 3.41a)

- Engage your core a little more strongly and allow the lower back to sink closer to the bale and begin to move the legs to the left, rolling more weight onto your left buttock and keeping the core working well to stop you rolling onto the floor. (Photo 3.41b)

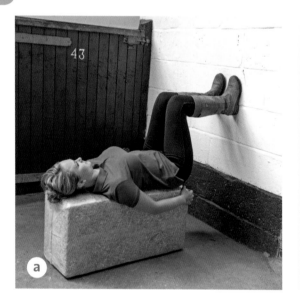
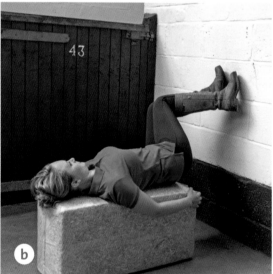

Photos 3.41a and b a) The neutral starting position with nice angles at the hip and knee.
b) Note how the core is engaged and the ribcage is still allowing only the lower back to rotate.

- Hold that position for a count of three, mentally scanning through your body for areas that may have tensed up; the shoulders perhaps?

- Return the body into the centre and then the legs. **Please note** that *the body must roll first* and then the legs follow. You could think about rolling the right buttock back onto the bale first, if that helps; the legs are attached to the pelvis so will follow anyway.

- Starting with the engagement of the core and the dropping of the lower back onto the bale, repeat the exercise to the other side.

> **Tip** I often ask clients to think of the movement coming only from the pelvis, to imagine that their pelvis is like the steering wheel of a car – to turn left, the left hip bone drops and the right hip bone lifts. If all the effort and emphasis is coming from the leg movement, the lower back will often arch away from the bale, which could cause discomfort.

Standing Chalk Circle

WITH THIS EXERCISE you are working to improve mobility in the back and stretching the arm, shoulder and neck muscles.

This is a lovely mobilisation and stretching exercise but **please note:** if you have a history of shoulder injury or dislocation it would be wise to check with your GP or health professional before commencing.

- Stand with your left side to a wall, in your neutral standing posture. Your arms are out in front of you, palms together, with the back of the left arm close to, or on, the wall. Your arms are roughly in line with the centre of your chest, no higher or your shoulders will shoot up by your ears! (Photo 3.42a)

- Imagine you are going to draw a circle around yourself with the right hand. Engage your core. Keeping the tips of the right fingers close to the wall move the right arm upwards, as the arm comes towards your head start to turn through your head and neck to keep looking at your arm. (Photo 3.42b)

- As you circle the arm further behind you, the fingers come away from the wall and the palm naturally turns outwards. Keep the rotation in your head and neck; your torso will also have begun to rotate, the chest turning outwards away from the wall. (Photo 3.42c)

- Once the arm comes roughly level with the underarm you rotate the arm so the palm again faces the wall, looking at the arm the whole time. Ensure your left hip is still in contact with the wall throughout and be aware that in your desire to move further you don't cheat and lean backwards from the lower back. Continue to circle the arm down and forwards, brushing the right thigh before returning to the starting position of palms together. (Photos 3.42d and e).

- Depending on how much time you have, circle the arm at least twice in that direction and then reverse the movement, circling the arm in the opposite direction, for the same number of repetitions.

- Turn around, establish your neutral standing posture and engage your core ready to repeat the exercise with the left arm, also in both directions.

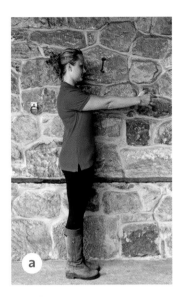

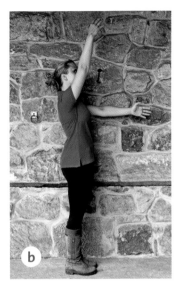

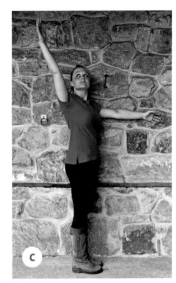

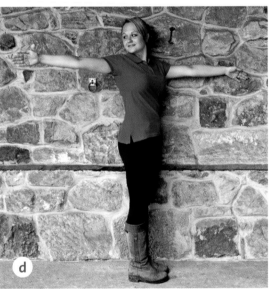

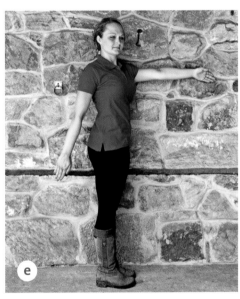

Photo 3.42a–e a)The starting position for the Chalk Circle. b) As the arm comes upwards the head and neck follow the movement. c) The arm starts to come behind Fay, who is doing a great job of keeping her pelvis and legs still. Note also the palm is starting to turn outwards now. d) Fay's shoulders are relaxed as the arm is fully behind her. e) Note the palm has turned inwards again as the arm comes toward the leg and returns to the starting position.

Tip I have yet to meet anyone who can keep their fingers on the wall throughout the whole circle without cheating and moving their body! Keep the pelvis and legs in their neutral starting position while you focus on getting a lovely even circle and stretch.

Standing Arm Openings

THIS IS A LOVELY rotational exercise to keep the back supple and is also a superb stretch for the front of the chest – great to help stretch out rounded shoulders.

- Stand in your neutral position with the left side of the body close to or touching a wall. Your arms are outstretched, keeping them roughly in line with the centre of your chest, certainly no higher or your shoulders will shoot up by your ears! Your palms are touching; the left arm is lightly in contact with the wall. (Photo 3.43a)

- Engage your core, and begin to take the right arm out to the side, turning through the head and neck as you do so; ensure your thumb stays in line with your nose (Photo 3.43b). Once your arm is fully out to the side and in line with the centre of your body, get that core working a little harder and start to rotate your back, starting from the top and working down, as the arm comes further behind you. The body is turning but the pelvis and legs stay facing forwards; visualise a pole in the centre of your spine that you are turning around to prevent you from leaning backwards. (Photo 3.43c)

- As you turn there are three things to watch out for.

  1. Ensure that it is only your back that has rotated/turned and that you have not leant backwards in an attempt to move further as this would put pressure on the small of your back.

  2. Keep the thumb in line with the nose even when you bring the arm behind you as we do not want you to over-stretch the shoulder.

  3. Keep the shoulders away from the ears.

- Begin to return the body and arm to the centre and then all the way back to the starting position. Repeat several times to that side before turning round to repeat the exercise with the left arm.

THE EXERCISES

Tip Do keep engaging your core throughout the exercise to support your back. You need to be very aware that the rotation of the torso doesn't include any leaning back; by taking time to feel that the weight is staying even across the whole foot and over both feet, i.e. you aren't leaning into one more than the other, as you rotate you should keep the spine in alignment and the hips facing forwards.

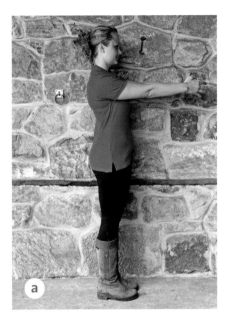

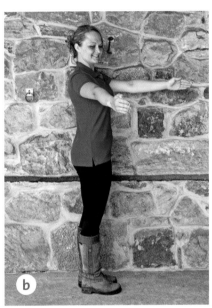

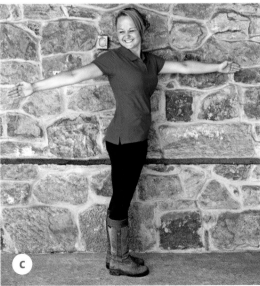

Photos 3.43a–c a)The neutral standing posture, arms out in front of you. b) As the arm moves to the centre, follow the movement with the head and neck. c) The arm is outstretched behind you but the pelvis stays facing forwards.

Rollbacks

THIS EXERCISE WILL really get the stomach muscles working and help to stretch the lower back – although you may actually just feel the tummy work during the exercise.

This exercise has been photographed using one bale of shavings but if you feel a little precarious make yourself a bigger surface with several bales, a large bale of hay, or just sit one bale in the centre of a nice deep stable bed – not that you are likely to fall off!

- Sit on the edge of your bale, legs in the 'chair' position as shown as this helps to keep your thighs from overworking and focuses the attention onto your stomach muscles. Hold your arms lightly out in front of you, slightly wider than shoulder-width apart. Keep the shoulders nice and relaxed. Feel that you are lengthening upwards through a relaxed back. (Photo 3.44a)

- You are going to take the back into a curved C-shape but do remember it is a *long* curve not a slump. Engaging your core, keep the shoulders and hips still and gently start to curve the whole back: imagine a big gym ball is being pressed into your torso and you are trying to mould your body around it. (Photo 3.44b)

- Take your focus to the back of the pelvis and gently start to roll the back of your trousers onto the bale starting from your tail bone (coccyx). Your whole body will start to move backwards.

- Really focusing on drawing those tummy muscles in, keep rolling your back down towards the bale, still focusing on the lower back moving more than the upper back – don't be tempted to push too hard into the mid-back thus changing your lovely curve into a hump back – the shoulders should be relaxed and don't hold your breath, keep breathing. (Photo 3.44c)

- Once you have rolled back into the last position shown (Photo 3.44d), hold the position as you take a breath and check that your thighs and buttocks haven't clenched. Then leading with the fingertips and the crown of your head, start to roll back up. Imagine someone is sitting behind you with their arms around your waist gently resisting you so that you keep that curve all the way forwards until your head is over your thighs. Once you have fully curved forward return to your upright sitting position ready to start again.

> **Tip** Start with smaller rollbacks to begin with as this is quite challenging for the abdominal muscles, if done correctly. You also need to be really, really vigilant that you are keeping your deep curve as you roll back to the start position as if you come up with a flat back you may strain your back.

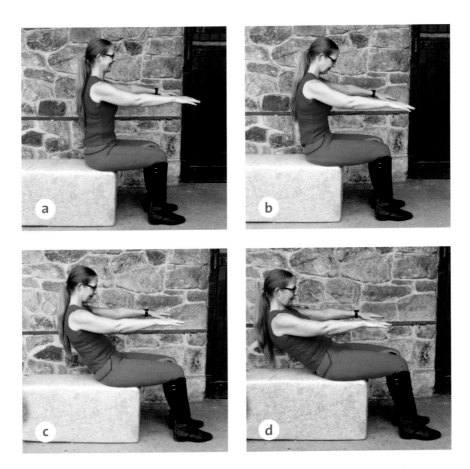

Photos 3.44a–d a) Sitting in a tall, neutral starting position. b) The body curves before you begin to roll back. c) Trying to roll the back of the pelvis down keeping a nice even curve – well done Jen! d) Taking the roll even further; Jen's face is still relaxed even though those tummy muscles are working really hard now.

Standing Back Extension

THIS EXERCISE introduces you to moving your spine into extension (bending backwards) which, although we don't do this during our everyday activities, is an important movement for overall back flexibility.

An important note before you begin: moving your back into extension is a good thing to do, it isn't something we do much of in our daily lives, however it is one Pilates exercise which can be done very badly, causing discomfort in the lower back. The reason it is done badly is that the lower back likes to bend backwards, and as such, people tend to only move from that area when they perform extension exercises. We need to get our backs moving much higher up, starting the movement from the top of the neck and only moving a little bit through each joint. This is a gentle stretch but it is very important to do it correctly.

- In the photos Jen is performing the exercise without support as our stable doors were too high but if you have something of the right height (something which comes slightly higher than waist height) you can stand against so that you can feel if the lower part of your back is misbehaving and moving that would be great.

- Stand in your neutral posture, weight evenly across your feet and core working lightly. Take one hand in the other and begin to raise the arms in front of your chest, shoulders relaxed and away from the ears. (Photo 3.45a) As the arms start to rise above nose level engage the core more firmly, lengthen up tall through your whole body as you start to gently curve your neck back slightly.

- Continue to move the arms upwards over your head and, one bone at a time, feel your back curving gently backwards. Your strong core will help to keep the lower part of your back still. (Photos 3.45b and c)

- Begin to lower the arms, returning your spine to neutral one bone at a time as you do so.

- Take a breath; I am sure you must have been holding it throughout the exercise because of the concentration.

> **Tip** Imagine you have a hand lightly placed on the lower back above your waist and another on the stomach. The area between the two hands has to stay completely still.

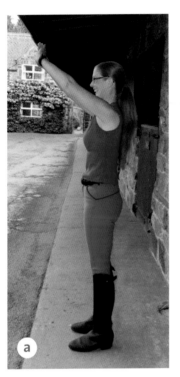
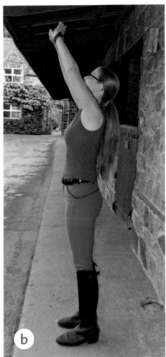
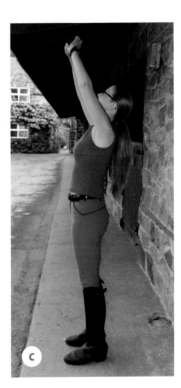

Photos 3.45a–c a) The arms come up, the shoulders stay down and the body stays in neutral. b) The extension starts with small movements from the base of the skull. c) Note the lower back has barely changed position as Jen has come fully back into extension.

Ribcage Closure

THIS IS A FAB shoulder and body-awareness exercise. It is particularly useful for isolating arm movements and becoming aware of the position of your ribcage and how it moves, or ideally doesn't move, when you raise your arms.

- You will need a lead rope, exercise stretch band, tail bandage or broom handle. This is to ensure your arms stay in the correct position throughout the exercise and will give you some visual feedback as to the level of your arms during the movements – you will see clearly if one hand is higher than the other as the rope will be on an angle.

- Sit on a bale or chair, feeling both seat bones are evenly weighted and that you are not rolling onto the back of your buttocks or forward onto your pubic bone – in other words, the pelvis is upright and neutral – and your spine has the correct neutral curves.

- Take hold of your rope with both hands, holding it slightly wider than shoulder-width apart. Lightly engage your core as you begin to raise the arms (but not the shoulders) until they are straight out in front of you. (Photos 3.46a and b)

- As you now continue to lift the arms higher (Photo 3.46c) you may feel that the front of the ribcage is also lifting and you are hollowing your back. If you cast your mind back to Chapter 2, this would mean that the imaginary light on your breastbone is now shining upwards. This is shortening the muscles in the lower back, which you do not want.

- Lower your arms again so that they are out in front of you and this time, as you begin to raise the arms up think about the bottom of your ribcage staying down, as if you were trying to tuck it lightly into the waistband of your trousers. You may feel more work going on in the tummy muscles now too. This is why the exercise is called Ribcage Closure: you are *closing* the ribcage downwards to keep the back in neutral.

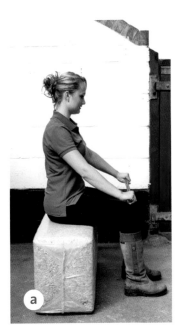 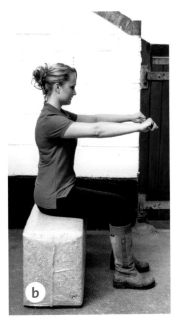 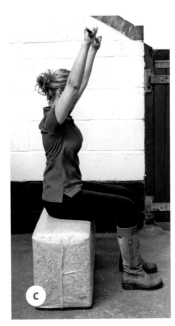

Photos 3.46a–c a) Arms in the starting position with the pelvis and spine in neutral. b) As the arms come up the shoulders stay down and relaxed. c) With the arms fully up, the body is still in neutral.

- Lower the arms all the way back to the start position and repeat. As the arms are lifting and lowering do keep checking that the hands, and thus the rope or band, are level; if you are stronger to one side you may pull that side more, lowering the rope to that side. This is also true if you are tighter in one shoulder.

Tip You may also use this exercise as a strengthening exercise for your shoulder stability muscles. As you bring your arms up in front of you and start to lift the arms higher, draw your shoulder blades down towards your waist and your underarms towards your hips – you should find that your arms do not go up as high with these muscles working. Do ensure you keep your ribs down throughout and keep an eye on the levelness of the rope as mentioned above.

Dumb Waiter

THIS SIMPLE EXERCISE will help to correct rounded shoulders by stretching the muscles at the front of the chest.

Please note that you must be careful with this exercise if you have dislocated your shoulder(s) in the past or had a recent shoulder injury.

- Sitting with your back in contact with a wall or door, ensuring you have the neutral curves to your spine, hold your forearms out in front, palms up as if holding a tray, with your upper arms in contact with your sides; elbows in contact with the wall and ideally in contact with your sides for the starting position. (Photo 3.47a)

- Engaging your core and keeping the upper arms and elbows in to your sides, take your forearms out to the side – think of your thumbs leading the movement. (Photo 3.47b) As you have taken the forearms wide, check that you haven't arched your back away from the wall; subconsciously you want to get the arms all the way to the wall but in doing so it is possible to cheat by arching your back and losing your neutral spine. Feel the stretch across the front of the chest, as though widening your collarbones.

- Once you have done one or two repetitions to get a feel for the movement you can now add in some strengthening work for your shoulder-stabilising muscles. With the arms out in front of you, be aware of where the outside edges of your shoulder blades are and using your back muscles, gently draw the shoulder blades down towards your waistband before you open the arms to the sides. By sitting against a wall you will feel this additional work in your back.

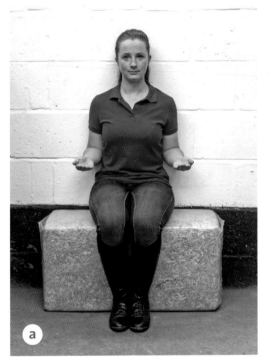 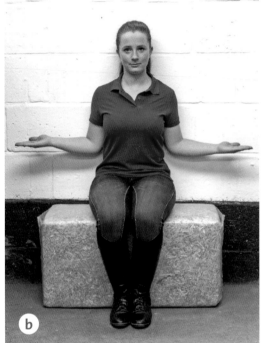

Photos 3.47a and b a) Arms out in the starting position.
b) The elbows stay on the wall as the arms open to the sides.

Standing Press-Up

THIS EXERCISE WILL strengthen the back of the arms (your triceps) and will help to improve your body awareness as you are required to keep your neutral standing posture as you perform the arm component of the exercise.

You may be wondering why there is an exercise in this book to strengthen the back of the arms but nothing for the front of your arms. If you think about everything you do on a daily basis, there's a lot of work already being done to keep the arms toned – lifting water buckets, haynets, sacks of feed – but few things work the triceps at the back of the upper arm. Until now...

- Stand facing a wall or door; to begin with stand an arm's length away from the wall. You are in your neutral standing posture with your core lightly engaged. (Photo 3.48a)

- Place your hands flat on the wall shoulder-width apart and slightly lower than the level of the tops of your shoulders. Engage your core a little more and begin to bend the elbows so you lean in towards the wall. Keep bending the elbows as you lower the forehead as close to the wall as you can (Photo 3.48b). As you bend the elbows make sure you maintain the following.

  - A lengthened, neutral body position – no bending in the middle, the bend comes from the ankle and elbows/shoulders only.
  - A strongly working core.
  - Most importantly, keep the elbows level with your sides, don't let them stick out like chicken wings. To get the work into the triceps the arms have to stay in line with the body.

At this point you might also be getting a lovely stretch in your calves too.

- Push yourself back to your upright standing position keeping the arms close to your sides so that you get the work in your triceps and, again, keeping your body in alignment as you do – don't let that middle bend!

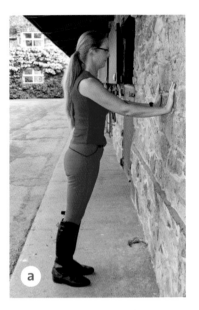

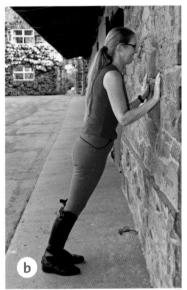

Photos 3.48a and b
a) The neutral starting position. b) Lean in to the wall with the elbows in to the sides ready to press back up; Jen is smiling as she knows this is the bit that will work the triceps.

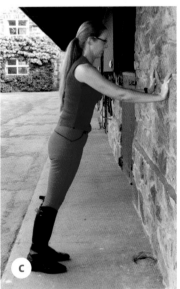

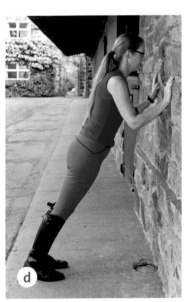

Photos 3.48c and d
c) Standing further away from the wall will work the triceps a bit more. d) Jen is not smiling now as this is really working her arms.

Windows

T HIS EXERCISE IS A favourite with clients; it really stretches the shoulders and chest increasing the mobility in the shoulder joint. It is a great exercise to improve your awareness of the ribcage position, thus improving your general posture.

Please note, this exercise takes your shoulders through a large range of movement so if you have a shoulder injury, please check with your GP or health professional that it is suitable for you to do.

There are four positions to this exercise and to make it easier to remember I have listed these positions followed by the detailed instructions.

- **Position 1: Arms up towards the sky** (Photo 3.49a) Lie on a bale with your spine and pelvis in neutral, knees bent and feet on the ground. Raise your arms up, pointing them towards the sky but keeping them slightly wider than shoulder-width apart and lengthen them lightly up; do not be tempted to push them up, which would cause tension in the shoulders and your chest to round forwards.

- **Position 2: Elbows out to the side** (Photo 3.49b) Engage your core and send your elbows out to the sides, still with the forearm and fingers pointing upwards. The elbows want to come down level with the sides of your body and keep them in line with your underarms; if they are higher it can make you feel tense and inclined to hunch your shoulders up.

- **Position 3: Rotate the upper arms so that your fingers point behind you** (Photo 3.49c) Engaging your core, while thinking of keeping the ribcage down and the back of the breastbone heavy, begin to rotate the upper arm so that your fingers now point behind you – as if you were surrendering.

- **Position 4: Stretch the arms behind you** (Photo 3.49d) With a little more core work and thoughts of keeping the front of the body heavy so you do not lift your back, stretch the arms behind you.

- Return the arms to the start position.

- The most important parts of this exercise are keeping your spine in neutral throughout and only working the arms within a comfortable range – you want to feel a stretch but don't break anything!

> **Tip** To increase the stretch, allow the elbows to drop further downwards (Position 2), but be aware that when you rotate them (Position 3), it is going to stretch more.

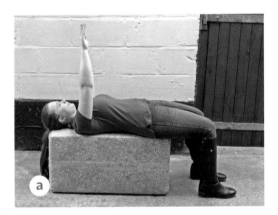
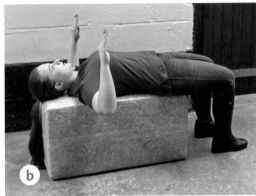
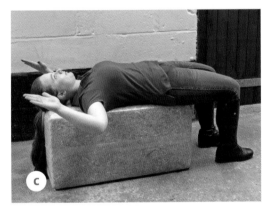
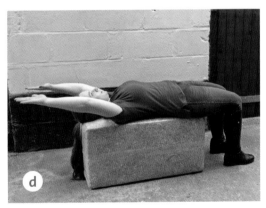

Photos 3.49a–d a) Position one. b) Position two. c) Position three. d) Position four.

Standing Quad Stretch

THE EXERCISES

T HIS IS A SIMPLE, do-anywhere stretch for the big muscles – the quads (quadriceps) – on the front of the thigh.

● In your strong, neutral standing posture bend one knee and take a hold of your foot or trouser leg. Keeping the supporting knee relaxed, gently draw the bent leg back until you feel a stretch down the front of the thigh. (Photo 3.50)

● Check you have not let your lower back dip or that you have tilted forwards. The leg you are stretching stays close to the supporting leg and should not wander off to the side.

● This is an important area to keep supple and stretched. Try to hold the stretch until you feel it begin to ease, rest out of the stretch for a count of three (still holding the foot) and then return the leg to a stretched position.

● Repeat to the other leg.

● If one leg is tighter than the other do a couple of extra stretches to the tighter side.

Please note you should not feel any discomfort in the knee of the leg you are stretching. If you do, use an alternative exercise: put a lead rope or similar band round the ankle and, keeping the knee joint at 90 degrees, think of pushing the thigh back.

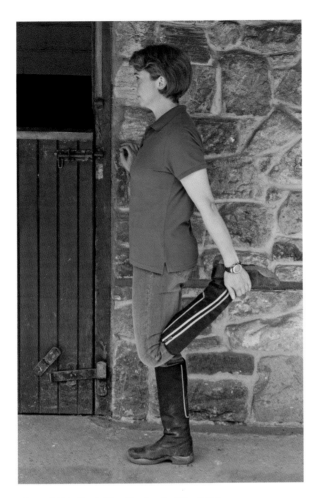

Photo 3.50 Stretching the front of the left leg.

Tip If you feel wobbly when doing the quad stretch, either hold onto something for support or hold onto your opposite ear lobe – for some reason this helps! This is such an important area to keep stretched so do it every time you fill water buckets, boil the kettle, wait for your horse to finish his feed etc.

Standing Hip Flexor Stretch

THIS IS A GREAT exercise for improving hip mobility by stretching the very top of the thigh. It also improves body awareness as you need to ensure you maintain your neutral torso position throughout to get the most benefit from the stretch.

- Stand with one leg resting on a bale as shown, then step forward with the supporting leg so that you are in a wide, stable stance (Photo 3.51a). Keeping your body upright with a neutral spine gently tuck your backside underneath you – think of your hip bones rolling back and your pubic bone coming forward (Photo 3.51b). As you do, take a little more weight in your supporting foot. You should feel a stretch in the front of the hip and/or top of the thigh.

- Hold the stretch for as long as is comfortable but don't rush it; this is an important area for horse riders to keep supple and free. As you are holding the stretch ensure your upper body is still in neutral, the temptation is to push the chest back and to slump.

- Repeat to the other side.

> **Tip** If you find you are feeling the stretch much further down the thigh, do the Standing Quad Stretch before this exercise.

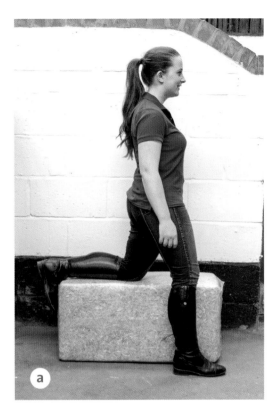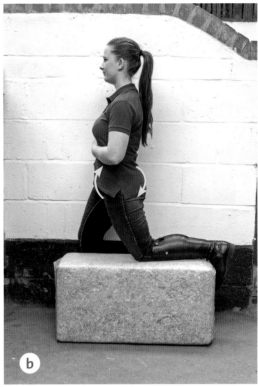

Photos 3.51a and b a) This view shows the forward position of the supporting leg.
b) A small roll of the pelvis (hip bones roll back slightly, pubic bone comes forward)
may be all you need to feel a stretch.

Lying Hip Flexor Stretch

AN EASY STRETCH for the very top of the thigh which will help with overall hip mobility – and you get to lie down while doing it!

- Without falling on the floor, sit with your buttocks just perched on the edge of a bale with your knees bent and feet on the floor. Take your left leg in towards you, hold onto it with one hand and use the other to hold onto the bale as you engage your core and slowly start to roll back until you are lying fully on the bale. You may now place both hands round the leg if you feel stable enough to do so.

- Check that your back is in neutral and focus particularly on keeping the lower back close to the bale so you don't over-arch it. Engage your core and slowly stretch your right leg along the floor until it is straight. You do need to keep engaging your core and keep the lower back down so as not to take any strain there, it will also help to deepen the stretch. (Photo 3.52)

- Slide the right leg back in again, rest for a moment and take the stretch again.

Photo 3.52 Note that Christie's lower back is down towards the bale, supported by her strong core.

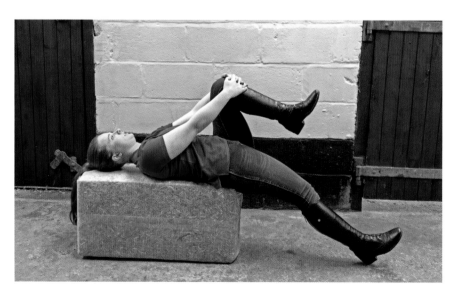

- To change to the other leg, firstly bring the right leg back to the starting position, engage your core and keep your lower back still as you lower the left leg down to the floor and bring the right in towards your chest.

Tip Getting out of this position without putting any strain on your back can be either easy or tummy challenging! The easy version is to try to roll onto your side (without falling off the bale) and sit up. The harder version is to bring both feet to the floor and roll up one bone at a time – practise your Rollback exercise first before doing this. Please **do not** thrust yourself upright by pushing the raised leg forward; that is horrible for your back!

Gluteal (Buttock/Backside Muscles) Stretch

THE EXERCISES

THIS SIMPLE STRETCH will help to keep these well-used muscles free from excessive tension. Due to the muscles' location around the back and sides of the pelvis, excessive tension can result in lower back pain and stiffness and hip mobility problems.

- This exercise has been demonstrated on a single bale of bedding; however, if you feel a little uneasy about falling off onto a hard floor then use a couple of bales or put the bale somewhere with a softer landing.

- Lying flat on the bale with your spine in neutral, bring your left leg in towards you and take hold of the back of the thigh with your left hand, using your right hand to balance on the bale if you need to. Engage your core but keep relaxed through your back and shoulders. Now bring your right leg in towards your chest and, almost as if you were going to cross your legs, place the outside of the right ankle over the left knee. If you feel comfortable doing so, place your right hand around the back of the left thigh too and pull the left leg in towards your chest more. (Photo 3.53)

- You should feel a stretch in your right buttock, possibly into the back of the right thigh, too. And if your hamstrings are tight, you may also get a stretch in the back of the left leg.

- To increase the stretch, draw the left leg in towards you. The feeling of the right knee pushing away from your chest may also change the stretch.

- If you feel you are straining your neck during this exercise place a folded sweater or jacket under your head.

- Repeat to the other side taking the time to only bring one leg in at a time to protect your lower back.

Photo 3.53 Both legs in position for the Gluteal Stretch. Make sure your neck stays relaxed throughout the exercise, particularly if you increase the stretch.

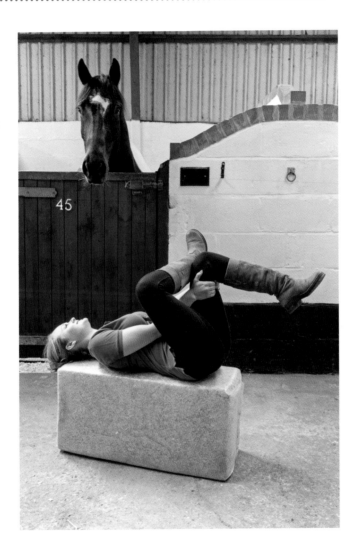

Lying Hamstring Stretch

THIS IS A REALLY effective stretch for the back of the thigh and the calf.

- You will need a stretch band, tail bandage, lead rope or similar for this exercise. Lying on a bale (or bales if you feel wobbly and prefer more surface to lie on) with your left foot on the floor for support, bend your right leg in towards you and put the bandage around your foot.

- Engaging your core and keeping your back in neutral, straighten the leg away from you, and then slowly pull it in towards you until you feel a stretch down the back of the leg.

- Hold the stretch – without holding your breath – until it begins to ease slightly, then lower the leg an inch or two, count to three and then bring the leg back in towards you until you feel a stretch again.

- Check that you are keeping your back in neutral and that your shoulders are relaxed, arms resting by your sides not pulling your leg in with all your might!

- Please do not judge how far your leg comes in by where the lovely Fay has hers in the photograph (Photo 3.54). Some of you may have very stretchy hamstrings and can get the leg in much further; some of you may struggle to get the leg as far as Fay. The more you do this exercise the easier it will become.

> **Tip** For an added stretch, bend your ankle so that your toes flex towards your nose – this will give you a gentle pull in your calf muscle. OK, I may have told a little white lie there – it may give you a **big** stretch in your calf.

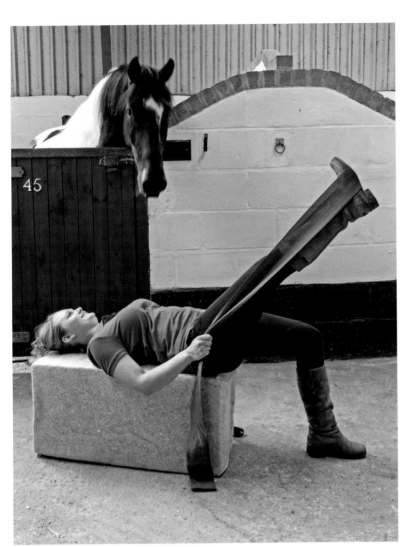

Photo 3.54 Only take the leg in as far as is bearable.

Inner Thigh Stretch

T**HIS REALLY IS A** very important stretch for horse riders; the inside thighs can become very tight so this stretch will help to keep the area flexible, which will help with hip mobility.

This is a very 'effective' stretch, and I must explain the use of 'effective' here. My lovely mat-work clients who have been with me for years got fed up with me telling them they were about to do a 'nice stretch' or a 'really good stretch' as they thought my definition of nice/good and theirs were poles apart, so they decided I was only allowed to use the word 'effective' – some may question who is in charge in my classes!

● Place a bale right next to a wall, with the short end on the wall. As elegantly as you can, roll onto your back and wriggle down until your buttocks are touching the wall; your legs should be straight, resting on the wall for support (Photo 3.55a).

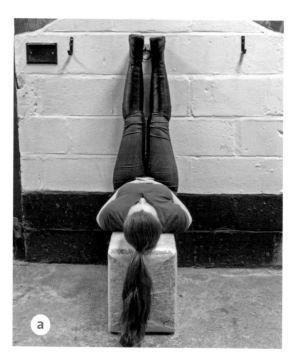

Photos 3.55a Try to start with your buttocks as close to the wall as you can.

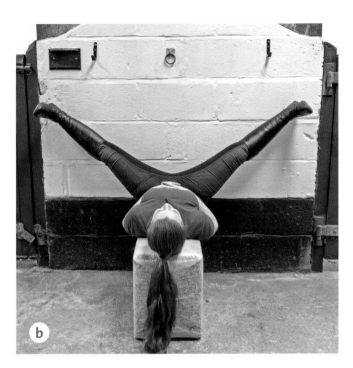

Photos 3.55b The finishing V-position of this stretch. Check the feet are level once you have reached the limit of your stretch.

- Ensuring your back and pelvis are in neutral, lightly engage your core and begin to slide the legs out into a V-position as shown (Photo 3.55b). Relax into that 'effective' stretch for as long as you can bear it. Take the legs back to the start position, have a short rest and then repeat.

- Keep scanning your body feeling for areas that may have tensed up – your jaw, face, shoulders, to name just a few.

Tip Once in your stretch and confident that you aren't likely to fall off your bale, have a look at your feet and see if they are level (see Photo 3.55b). It is likely that one foot will be slightly higher than the other so keep a note that this is your stiffer side and try to release more to that leg, but do it gradually! I do not want to hear of any groin strains!

Calf Stretch

THE CALF MUSCLES are connected to both the ankle and knee area; two important joints for absorbing the movement of the horse when we ride. Keeping these areas supple will make riding more comfortable and stable.

- Stand facing a door or wall, roughly an arm's length away, and place your palms on the wall just below shoulder height. Engage your core and take a step back with your right leg. Push the right heel lightly to the floor as you bend the left knee and lean, from the ankles only, towards the wall until you feel a stretch in the right calf.

- You must ensure that as you have leant in you have maintained the line from ear, shoulder, centre of ribcage, hip, knee to ankle (Photo 3.56); don't dip in the middle or stick your buttocks in the air.

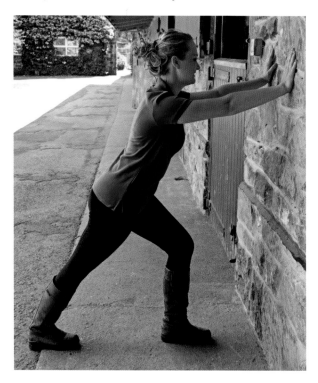

Photo 3.56 Fay is keeping a nice line from her ear through to her ankle.

- Lift the right heel, rest for a count of three, and then press the heel back to the floor. If the stretch has eased you may step back a little further.

- Step in to the start position and repeat with the left leg.

> **Tip** It is difficult to tell you precisely how far to step back as all of us have varying degrees of flexibility in our calves. To be on the safe side, start with a smaller stretch and increase it as your muscle flexibility improves.

Cherry Picking

A GOOD EXERCISE for maintaining and improving mobility in the feet and ankles.

This great little exercise is so good for keeping your feet and ankles supple; however, it does have the side-effect of inducing the most awful cramp sometimes, so you have been warned! It may also be one exercise best done without footwear so perhaps one for a quiet moment of rest before or after a ride?

- You may do this exercise in a seated or lying position; if lying on your back hold on to the back of your thigh to support the leg with your ankle in a relaxed, neutral position. Imagine you are picking cherries from a tree but you have to use your toes not hands.

- **Position 1: The start position** (Photo 3.57a).

- **Position 2: Grasp the cherries** Stretch the front of the ankle so that you point your foot away from you, then curl the toes underneath your foot as if grasping a cherry or two (Photo 3.57b).

- **Position 3: Collect the cherries** Hold onto that fruit with the toes as you bend the ankle bringing the top of the foot in towards you (Photo 3.57c).

- **Position 4: Drop the cherries** Rotate the ankle so the foot points inwards and open the toes, dropping your imaginary cherries. Repeat the exercise but this time when you bring your cherries back in, rotate the foot and drop them to the outside (Photo 3.57d).

- Repeat several times in each direction before changing to the other foot.

> **Tip** This exercise is very good for working the muscle along the outside of the shin. If, however, the cramp becomes unbearable you could do some ankle circles instead.

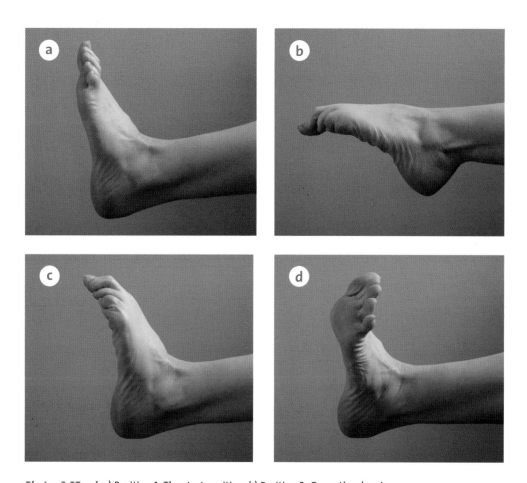

Photos 3.57a–d a) Position 1: The start position. b) Position 2: Grasp the cherries. c) Position 3: Bending the ankle to bring the top of the foot towards you. d) Position 4: Rotate outwards and drop the cherries.

EQUESTRIAN PILATES FOR
EVERYDAY YARD TASKS

4

I am hopeful that having read the previous chapters you will already be thinking differently about how you use your body in almost everything you do. So many people come to me saying that their back/shoulder/hips etc. are painful or uncomfortable when they ride but as I watch them walking, sitting or even taking their shoes off it is obvious that those areas are tight and/or out of alignment off the horse and that it is the act of trying to sit nicely upright and squarely in the saddle that is causing the discomfort. When they are off the horse they are free to be as twisted and uneven as they like, as the office chair or surface they walk on isn't likely to stick its ears back and complain! Does that make sense?

The jobs we do around the stable yard to make sure our beloved equine is warm, clean, comfortable, well fed and watered are some of the tasks most likely to wreak havoc on our bodies. For example, hands up anyone who has picked up a bale of bedding with ease and carried it to the stable? Nobody? Well, hands up those who have managed to get their arms around a bale of bedding and waddled in the most ungainly manner to the stable, stopping occasionally to correct the inevitable 'Aargh! I'm about to drop it' moment? Yes, me too!

Lifting bedding or bales of hay is one of those jobs that unless you are very tall, with very long arms and very big muscles, you cannot really do correctly. In putting this book together I have tried, with the photographer, to look at all possible methods and really the only safe way of handling these bulky items is to use a sack-trolley or wheelbarrow or for two people to lift them together. If you have no option but to move them without assistance, concentrate on engaging your core and shoulder stabilisers before you proceed.

There are, however, other stable yard jobs I *can* help with.

SWEEPING

Excuse my hideous over-acting in Photo 4.1 but I was trying to mimic the main faults I see. Firstly you will see that I am using quite a lot of effort with my upper shoulder muscles and neck, my upper trapezius in particular; my shoulders are up by my ears and I am taking quite a bit of strain through my arms. I have automatically stepped forward to push off with my favoured leg – we all have one! The other thing to note is my back is rather hunched – no sign at all of the neutral curves – and I can tell you that there was no core working. If you compare the photos you may also notice that I am taking my weight backwards in Photo 4.1 but in Photo 4.2 my posture is more upright, my core is engaged and I have stepped forward with my 'unfavoured' leg. Because we *do* all have one side we favour, the more we submit to the use of this side over the other the more wonky we will become. If you look at Photo 4.1 you can see clearly that the pelvis is twisted.

Think about how often you sweep, muck out and push wheelbarrows (and do other non-horse-related activities like walking up stairs) then it doesn't take long to become very one-sided. It will take time to get used to using the other leg as you will have to consciously choose it and build up the muscle memory to become proficient at using the other side of the body. I should also state the obvious, which is: once you have got used to using the other leg, remember to alternate between the two or you will end up swapping one favoured leg for another!

The other point to note in Photo 4.2 is my shoulder position. I have now drawn my shoulders down as described earlier in the section on

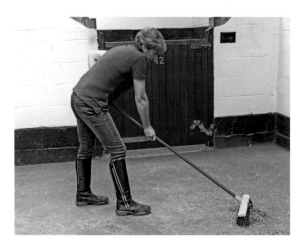

Photo 4.1 How not to sweep.

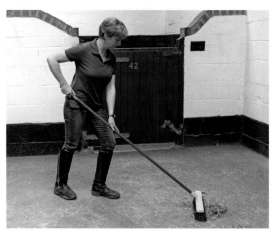

Photo 4.2 A better sweeping posture.

Shoulder Stability (page 30). All in all, this is not only a more comfortable way to sweep but it is more efficient. Instead of using small muscle groups, like those in the arms, neck and shoulders, you can get those big, powerful back, leg and core muscles working. Notice how I am leaning more forward in Photo 4.2, using the weight of my body to sweep rather than exhausting my arms.

MUCKING OUT

As with sweeping, the over-use of shoulders, neck and arms is very apparent in Photo 4.3. You will also see that the back position is hunched, no core muscles are working and I am again leading with my favourite leg. If you are mucking out a particularly wet and/or dirty bed you do not need me to tell you that it can be heavy work and if you are just using the smaller muscles of the arms, shoulders and neck rather than getting the larger back and core muscle groups involved, you will soon tire.

In Photo 4.4 you will note the more neutral body and shoulder position. I have again changed the leading leg and have also swapped arms – a good habit to get into; the more you practise the easier it will become. Note the whole body is now involved in the activity; by taking the weight into the front foot I can take the effort away from just the shoulders and arms.

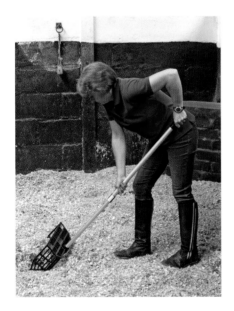

Photo 4.3 A bad mucking-out posture.

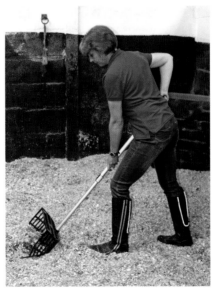

Photo 4.4 A good mucking-out posture.

PUSHING WHEELBARROWS

Oh, this is my favourite thing to nag clients about. I am so conscious of it I had real trouble doing the bad pose for Photo 4.5. What am I talking about? Those of you who 'carry' your wheelbarrow rather than push it – you know who you are! You insist on lifting the handles so high that the benefits of having a wheelbarrow are lost because you are using so much shoulder and arm work you might as well be carrying a large bucket – badly!

As you will also see in Photo 4.5, there is often a tendency to stoop when you are pushing and not engage the core. As with the previous activities, the favoured leg is leading the task and, because this is generally a heavier activity, then it is even more important to change.

When you are pushing your wheelbarrow think about all of the cues for your good standing posture: neutral spine, neutral pelvis, engaging your core. As you bend to take hold of the handles, ensure you bend from the knees and hips rather than hunching through the small of your back, and engage the core a little more strongly as you push upright through the legs to take the weight of the barrow. Also, draw the shoulder blades down and in towards your waistband as you take the weight as this should stop you from lifting with top of the shoulders and the neck. Finally, remember which leg to step forward with first to ensure your favoured leg doesn't do all of the work.

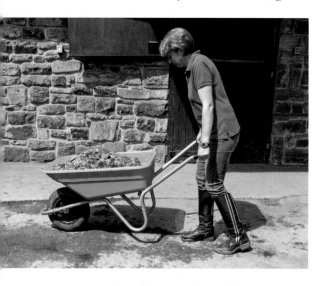

Photo 4.5 Bad wheelbarrow pushing; the barrow is being 'carried'.

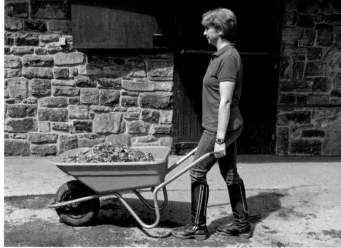

Photo 4.6 Good wheelbarrow pushing; the body is being used correctly to push rather than carry the barrow.

CARRYING BUCKETS AND HAYNETS

I have grouped these two tasks together as they have one common element, which is: we often carry the offending items on one side only. We either lean our body away from the item we are carrying to counter-balance the weight of the item, or we allow ourselves to tip toward the weight. (Photos 4.7 and 4.8) Either way, if this is repeated day after day we will eventually become tighter and shortened to one side.

Before picking up your bucket or haynet, engage your core. As you bend to pick it up, bend the knees and keep your back as neutral as possible. Push yourself upright using the leg muscles, engaging the core more as you take the weight of the item. Once upright, holding your net or bucket, check that you haven't allowed the tops of the shoulders to overwork. (Photos 4.9 and 4.10)

With haynets I often see people holding the cord diagonally across the body, using it as an extra tool to help carry the burden. You could try what I do and tie the end of the cord halfway down the net so that you have a strap you can put over your shoulder (see Photo 4.10). Even this is not ideal as you are still loading one side only but it is better than the alternative.

I hope that you are now starting to see that the bad and good ways to do your yard tasks are quite similar across a wide range of jobs.

Bad = over-use of shoulders, poor back posture, no core working, favouring one side.

Good = use of shoulder stabilising muscles, maintaining a neutral spine where possible, always starting a task with the conscious thought of engaging your core (especially if it is heavy work), alternating your favoured leading leg.

OTHER DAILY TASKS

When looking after a horse there are so many repetitive tasks involved (grooming, picking out hooves, leading, leaning over feed bins, etc.) that I could fill many more pages with tips. However, as we have already seen in this chapter the more you think about how you use your body well, the stronger and more able you will be to continue carrying out these tasks for years to come. Check that you are doing the following.

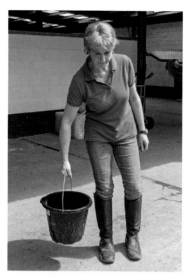

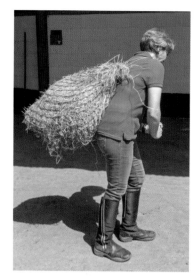

Photo 4.7 *far left* Bad bucket carrying – I am tipping towards the weight putting strain on my back.

Photo 4.8 *left* Bad haynet carrying – my shoulders and back are hunched and I am bracing away from the weight of the haynet.

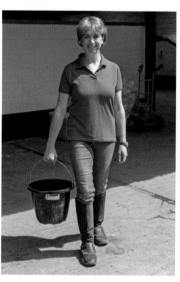

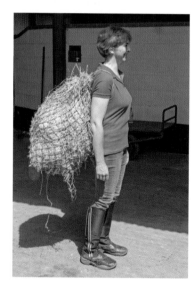

Photo 4.9 *far left* Good bucket carrying – a lovely upright posture, shoulder stabilisers and core working well.

Photo 4.10 *left* Good haynet carrying – a lovely upright posture, shoulder stabilisers and core working well and by looping the haynet over my shoulder I am not bracing away from the weight.

- Using your core muscles.
- Keeping your posture as neutral as the task will allow.
- Ensuring your shoulder stabilisers are working and that raised shoulders (shoulders up by your ears) are a thing of the past.
- Alternating your push-off (leading) leg.
- Working your arms equally.
- Using your wheelbarrow as a wheelbarrow.
- Making use of a big, strong giant to carry your bedding!

EQUESTRIAN PILATES
IN THE SADDLE

5

I have tuition from two riding instructors; the results they are working towards are the same but they are often presented differently. To that end, it is impossible for me to know how you were taught (perhaps you were self-taught) or are presently being taught by your instructor, nor your individual aims and aspirations and, indeed, the areas you find challenging. What I will offer you here are some ideas on how to use the Equestrian Pilates techniques in relation to your riding and common riding faults.

YOUR WARM-UP

Actually, this is *my* warm-up but I am a generous person and happy to share it! You now have a toolbox of exercises from the earlier chapters that you can use to warm yourself up physically before you get on your horse, selecting the exercises most beneficial to your body and needs.

When I get on Ari, to school him or hack out, I try to take the time to mentally and physically make the change from 'Sue, dashing round on two feet' to 'Sue, perfectly mouldable extension to Ari on four feet'. Although I want to be able to have an effect on him when I need to, a change of gait or rein for example, the rest of the time I want to interfere as little as possible with his natural balance and athleticism. This is how I recommend you warm up in walk.

- Relax and release. Take nice, slow breaths and on every out-breath focus on releasing any areas of tension in the whole body, becoming more and more relaxed with each breath.

- Feel the legs becoming softer and heavier, allowing the thighs to almost melt downwards. As the thighs become heavier the knees lengthen downwards, which allows the lower leg to become relaxed and free. Let the feet lightly rest on the stirrups.

- With the feeling of the legs still lengthening downwards, focus your attention on your seat, feeling that you are sitting evenly on both seat bones. The buttock muscles are relaxed; the hips are becoming more and more released.

- Feel the horse's ribcage moving beneath you, allowing it to rock your legs from side to side as it swings. Do you feel you are moving freely and evenly on both sides? Can you release more in the hips and legs?

- As the horse's hind leg steps under him feel how your seat is moved; lifted on one side, lowered on the other. Does this feel smooth and even? Are you able to relax your lower back and buttock muscles further to allow this movement to become even smoother?

- Maintaining the feeling of released hips and legs, return your attention to your seat. How heavily are you sitting? Could you be lighter? Imagine your saddle has become very fragile and delicate; starting with the lower part of your tummy, begin to engage your core, checking as you do that you have not over-engaged other muscles in the legs, buttocks and hips. Now feel the core is drawing upwards, almost under the ribcage to help you lighten away from your delicate saddle.

- Continue that feeling of 'upwards' through your relaxed spine, imagine someone running their finger up your back, all the way up to your neck and head. Feel as though someone has cupped your head in their hands and is softly drawing you skyward.

- As the spine is lengthening up, the shoulders, torso and arms remain soft and relaxed – like a soft cashmere jumper hanging from a padded coat-hanger: the skeleton is the hanger, the body is the jumper moulding gently around it. (See Photo 5.1)

- And now begin to ride . . .

What I notice time and time again is that by running through this exercise, the horse becomes as relaxed, released and focused as the rider. Record the above exercise onto an MP3 or phone and listen to it (only if safe to do so) so that you can remember your warm-up perfectly.

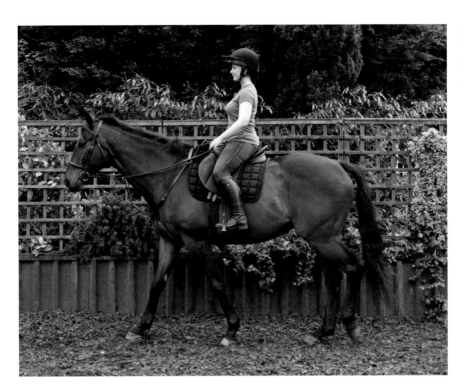

ROUNDED SHOULDERS

The shoulders hunching or rounding forward is quite common on and off the horse (Photo 5.2 overleaf). Many of us have to work on computers and drive cars, activities that exacerbate this problem. Many a riding instructor will simply ask you to 'push your shoulders back', but this does not help. If anything, it fixes one problem but causes another. If you sit with your back up against a chair or wall and allow your shoulders to round forwards can you feel that your back loses some neutral curves? Now, if you push your shoulders back can you feel how your back has curved the other way, chest lifting away from the wall and lower back shortening? You may also feel quite tense between the shoulder blades.

Return to your rounded shoulder position. Take your focus to where your shoulder blades are on your back, particularly the outside edge of the shoulder blades. Gently, using your back muscles, begin to slide your shoulder blades downwards and very, very slightly inwards. Did you feel how that opened up the front of the chest, bringing the shoulders back into position and the spine back into neutral?

Photo 5.2 Christie deliberately slumps her shoulders forward and braces her legs – notice how grumpy Jack looks about it!

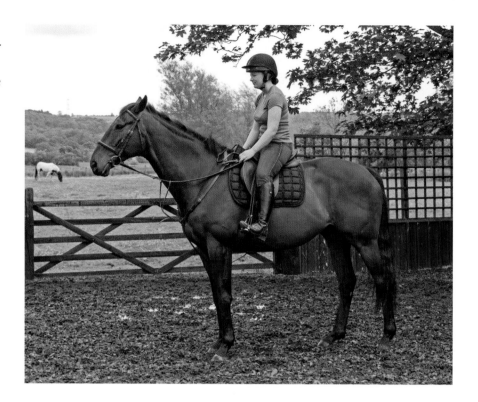

TIPPING FORWARDS

There are several reasons why riders tip forwards (Photo 5.3). The most common one I come across is where the rider's hip flexor muscles, i.e. the psoas and iliopsoas muscles (search the internet for images of these muscles; the way they work is fascinating), which broadly run from the lower back to the top of the thigh become tight and over-enthusiastic, by which I mean that the hip flexors take over the role of the stabilising muscles from transversus abdominis, the main core muscle.

The hip flexors bend you in the middle: if you are standing and bring your leg up into your knee-fold position (see page 50), that is your hip flexor working. If you keep the legs straight and bend forward from the hip/top of the thigh, that also is your hip flexor. So if you are riding and become unbalanced but also want to keep the legs still and in position, if you use the hip flexors rather than the transversus core muscle in an attempt to rebalance yourself, they will pull you forward. Likewise if you are gripping tightly with the legs the only other part of you that can move is your trunk, so you tip forward.

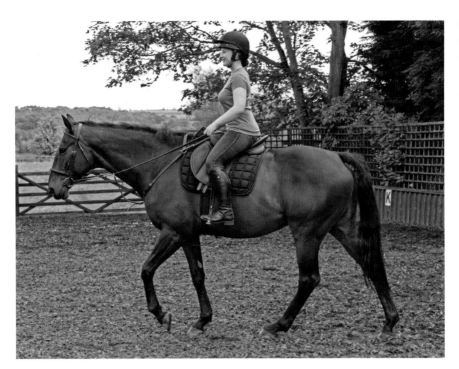

Photo 5.3 Christie is trying to demonstrate tipping forwards but it is not easy for her well-schooled body.

Learning to stretch and release the hip flexors using the exercises in Chapter 3 combined with strengthening and isolation of your core and improving your balance and stability, should all help to prevent you tipping forwards.

KNEES LIFTING

We have already discussed in the previous section how the hip flexors can take on the role of stabilising muscles, and the knees lifting up is another example of muscle groups overworking and/or taking the sta-bilising role. The more you can keep in your mind the sensation of the thighs softly lengthening, almost melting down, the less likely you are to over-use the big thigh muscles and to allow the legs to creep up. If, on the other hand, you think about 'pushing' the legs down, can you feel how that is a completely different sensation? It induces tension in the legs – we do need muscle tone in our legs to ride, but not tension.

Another tip to prevent the leg creeping up is to imagine you have an elasticated tail bandage tied round one thigh, it goes round the horse's backside and is then tied around the other thigh, just tight enough to draw the legs back slightly. That feeling of the legs drawing back will help to keep your seat deep, thus making you feel more stable. Notice I did not tell you to *push* the legs back; try it, it will give you a completely different sensation likely to make you feel very unstable!

SITTING TO ONE SIDE

No matter how hard we try, none of us will ever be truly balanced, even a Pilates instructor! Some riders do sit very obviously over to one side and it is one of the trickiest problems to unpick. There could be three things at fault:

1. The rider is crooked.

2. The horse is crooked.

3. The saddle is crooked.

There can also be a combination of all three problems and I will use myself as an example. Nearly three years ago I badly damaged my left shoulder slipping on ice. For around two years I didn't think I would ever be able to teach Pilates again as, even after surgery, it was excruciatingly painful. During that time, wallowing in self-pity, I let my guard down and subconsciously began over-using my right lower back and buttock muscles, resulting in me becoming very right-side dominant and it has taken a long time to fix.

Two years ago my horse sustained an injury to his left shoulder, and he too began to use his right hind leg and right-side quarters to compensate, again something we have had to work hard to rebalance.

One year ago I bought a second-hand treeless saddle and pad, which was also slightly worn on the left front/right rear diagonal. I didn't notice this until I scrutinised it. The result? My bulging disc problem returned as a result of the shortening and over-use of my lower back on one side, Ari became grumpy about being ridden because he was sore and the saddle pad ended up in the rubbish! The moral? Always look at the whole picture to solve this problem of sitting to one side; in my case all three possible faults could have individually or collectively caused the problem.

If the rider is at fault, the seated back exercises in Chapter 3 will help to both identify and release your tighter side. It is also worth working through the hip exercises as they too will identify and release imbalances. This may sound strange, but I have had many a client who has had one buttock more developed than the other (yes, I do mean one buttock can be bigger than the other), which will *definitely* knock you off balance. Lots of one-leg Pilates Stance Pliés are prescribed for that issue.

One of the most illogical things you may be asked to do in the saddle if you do sit to one side is to put more weight into the other seat bone. As the photos here show, all this will do is make you even more crooked (Photos 5.4a and b). If you are aware that you take more weight to one side try and think about the opposite thigh lengthening downwards. This will gently readjust your seat.

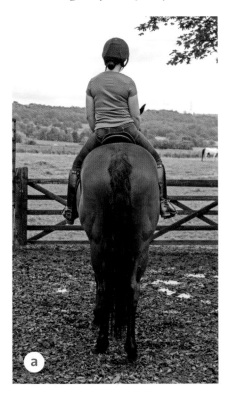 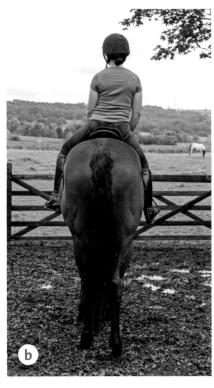

Photos 5.4a and b
a) Christie sitting to one side. b) This is what happens if she tries to sit more on her other seat bone: the curve in her back has increased.

A FINAL THOUGHT

Often it is the words an instructor chooses when trying to help that cause as many problems as they are aiming to fix. The following are common examples of poor instructions.

- **Heels down** Result: the leg braces and shoots forwards.

- **Sit up tall** Result: the chest sticks out and up with the lower back tensing and shortening.

- **Shoulders back** Result: the ribcage lifts forwards with the lower back over-arching.

- **Push with the seat** Result: everything tenses.

Always try to have in mind your neutral positions, your strong core and the sense of lengthening your body but staying grounded through your feet and seat. The more you are able to be relaxed and released in your riding, the less effort you will have to put into it: your aids will be heard clearly by your horse because the rest of your body will be quiet.